THE HISTORY OF
DOMESTIC
PLANT
MEDICINE

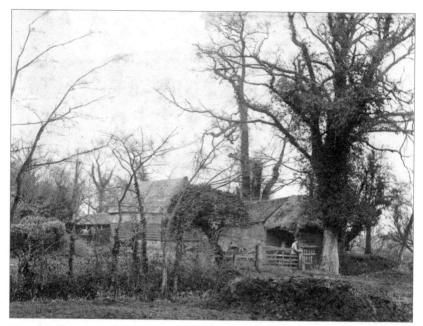

Farm buildings in Suffolk, from an album possibly by Clutterbuck. (© Norfolk Rural Life Museum)

THE HISTORY OF
DOMESTIC
PLANT
MEDICINE

GABRIELLE HATFIELD

Front cover images: Nicholas Culpeper, *The Complete Herbal* (1842).
(Royal College of Physicians, London/Wellcome Collection)

First published 1999
This paperback edition first published 2022

The History Press
97 St George's Place, Cheltenham,
Gloucestershire, GL50 3QB
www.thehistorypress.co.uk

British Library Cataloguing in Publication Data.
A catalogue record for this book is available from the British Library.

ISBN 978 1 80399 190 0

Typesetting and origination by The History Press
Printed and bound in Great Britain by TJ Books Limited, Padstow, Cornwall.

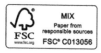

Trees for LYfe

CONTENTS

Preface to the New Edition

In the twenty-three years since the publication of this book, nearly all the people in East Anglia and throughout the country who shared their knowledge of plant remedies with me have died and, as far as I know, they had not passed on these remedies to others. I feel very fortunate to have had access to these last vestiges of country remedies. Today, passing through the villages and hamlets where these people lived, I reflect on how hard their lives were, contending with sometimes grinding poverty and no access to medical care, at least when they were children.

I remember a visit to an old lady who lived in a small, crooked cottage on a hillock in a small rural common. In her front garden there was a well, with watercress growing out of the top. Innumerable cats were prowling around and, when I approached the front door, some wound their way around my legs. It seemed like the beginning of a children's fairy tale.

But the story of the old lady's childhood was a nightmare, not a fairy story. She eventually escaped a cruel upbringing when she inherited the cottage from an aunt and came to live in it. The lady told me that her aunt knew the uses of every wild plant on the common, but that she only remembered a few – one was the use of vervain (*Verbena officinalis*) for sunburn. I asked her what she did if her cats were ill. 'Oh, I give them comfrey. If the hens are looking poorly, I give them comfrey; if the geese aren't laying, I give them comfrey,' she replied. When I left, she insisted on giving me a large bunch of watercress and two enormous white goose eggs.

Nowadays, as fewer and fewer of our large population have good access to the countryside and less and less of the countryside remains unpolluted, it would be hard to have such self-reliance, even if we wanted it. Yet these human stories from the recent past hold valuable lessons for us still today. We are beginning to realise that it is not necessary to travel to the rainforest for lost medicinal remedies; many of our own native plants will repay pharmacological studies. Such studies are difficult and expensive, but nevertheless will prove worthwhile, and vestiges of knowledge of their historical usage can be used as pointers to those species that may prove especially beneficial.

And maybe, just maybe, we could all benefit from practising a little more of the self-reliance that was forced upon the rural poor in the past. Perhaps, we could then be less dependent on our over-stretched NHS.

Gabrielle Hatfield, 2022

LIST OF ILLUSTRATIONS

ACKNOWLEDGEMENTS

I am grateful to the Author's Foundation for financial support when I began this book; to the Wingate Trust for a two-year Scholarship, and for their help and encouragement; to librarians and archivists, especially in Edinburgh and Norwich, for their patient help over many years; to Elizabeth Stratton, archivist at the John Innes Centre, for her help with the illustrations. I would like to thank the numerous individuals who have shared their memories and knowledge with me.

The Rudyard Kipling quotation from *Rewards and Fairies* (p. 15) is reproduced by permission of A.P. Watt on behalf of the National Trust, and extracts from *A Countryman's Day Book* are reproduced by permission of J.M. Dent/The Orion Publishing Group Ltd.

Finally, I wish to thank my publishers for their help, support and encouragement, and John, Amanda, Sarah, Clare and Jonathan for their love and patience and for keeping my sense of humour alive.

PICTURE CREDITS

I am grateful to the Biggar Museum Trust for permission to reproduce the photograph on page 181 (Janet Bell). The illustration on page 178 (Adam of Bethelnie) is reproduced by Permission of the Trustees of the National Library of Scotland. I would like to thank Stella Ross-Craig, the Royal Botanical Gardens, Kew, and the John Innes Foundation Historical Collections for the plant illustrations.

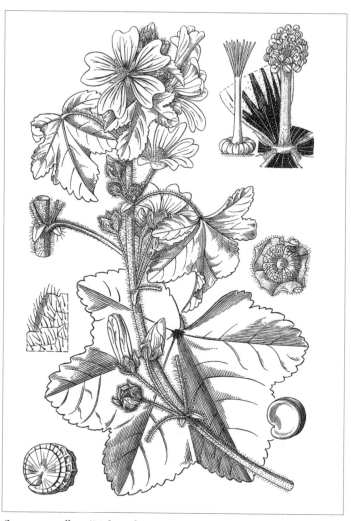

Common mallow (*Malva sylvestris*), from Stella Ross-Craig, *Drawings of British Plants.* (By kind permission of the Royal Botanical Gardens, Kew/photograph courtesy of John Innes Foundation Historical Collections)

INTRODUCTION

Anything green that grew out of the mould
Was an excellent herb to our fathers of old.
Rewards and Fairies
Rudyard Kipling

The story I wish to tell in this book concerns the use in
Britain of everyday plants for treating everyday ailments,
and it is the history of self-help rather than of official
medicine. For early man, plants were the most obvious
source of food, and their use in treating illnesses was
probably discovered incidentally. Such discoveries would
have obvious importance, and would be passed down from
one generation to the next. Once written records began,
some of this knowledge began to be recorded, but such
recording was, by definition, done by the educated sector
of society. The ordinary person would continue to use the
knowledge passed down to him orally from his forebears.
Little by way of written information would have filtered
through to the mass of society. For this reason, a study of
the history of medicine based on written records must be

skewed heavily in favour of the medicine preached and practised by the educational elite. This book is an attempt to redress the balance, and to give some account of the ordinary do-it-yourself medicine practised by the ordinary person in Britain.

Yet if there is no written record of what is primarily an oral tradition, how can we hope to reconstruct the humble home medicine of the past? We have to rely on fragments of information available in poetry, proverbs, songs and ballads, all of them products of oral traditions. In addition, we can obtain snippets of information from the writings of the literate, on the occasions on which they refer to the practices of their uneducated countrymen. Another source of information may come as more of a surprise. It is still possible, though only just, to obtain information from country people in Britain concerning plant remedies used by them within living memory. Some of these remedies show a quite astonishing story of continuity through the generations. An example will illustrate this. While talking to a man in his sixties, now resident in Norfolk, it emerged that he was brought up in Scotland by his elderly grandmother, herself a great believer in simple plant remedies. He vividly remembered stories she had told him as a child of her own great-grandmother, whose family survived unscathed a fever that wiped out most of her village. The explanation given was that the house was 'all hung about with onions', and onions were also used as food. The outbreak of fever must have occurred some time during the eighteenth century, yet this story was being told as vividly as if it were a recent occurrence. Moreover, the message of eating onions to combat infection was still very firmly practised in the family, as indeed it is in many areas of Britain. Incidentally, this use of onions is now being vindicated by modern pharmacology.

Allowing for poetic exaggeration, Rudyard Kipling's claim quoted at the beginning of this introduction was probably quite accurate. The word 'herb', although in botanical terms restricted to those green plants which die down in the winter, has in the past been used to signify all those plants useful to man, and it is in this broad sense that the term will be used throughout this book. In the past, herbs have for instance been used in food, perfumery, cosmetics, preservation of food and of the dead, as well as in medicine and contraception. Plants were the most obvious food source for early man, and in the days of pre-history their use in food and medicine were probably indistinguishable at first. Gradually it would have been found that certain food plants had medicinal properties, and trivial daily ailments would have been self-treated. As the recognition of serious illness began, the need for healers arose. Arguably, man used to self-treat with plants only the less serious and less mysterious illnesses, and these were treated by common-sense use of plants empirically found to be effective. However, desperate diseases need desperate remedies. The distinction must always have been apparent between, for example, accidental injury and more mysterious progressive disease such as TB or cancer. This distinction may have given rise to the need for healers; and the lore, myth, mystery and superstition so often quoted as part of traditional medicine may in fact have arisen not around self-medication with plants but around the healers and their healing rituals. This idea is discussed in the following chapters.

The history of domestic medicine in Britain has been largely ignored, apart from the Victorian and somewhat patronizing account by W.G. Black.[1] Much has been written about the recorded plant medicines of the herbals, and of the herbalists, but these records omit some of the everyday plant medicines used by our forebears. The subject matter of this book is an account of a neglected part of our national heritage, and as such has its own intrinsic interest. The use of our common native British plants in everyday home medicine is now almost obsolete: it is a matter of urgency to record the knowledge of such plant usage for posterity. The distilled wisdom of the centuries is something that we should proudly preserve, rather than patronizingly dismiss. There is an urgent need to conserve such knowledge of plant usage, before, like the rainforest, it has disappeared irrevocably. It is hoped that this book might provide some pointers to serious students of ethnobotany, and lead to the thorough investigation of more of our native British plants, and to the rediscovery of some of their forgotten medicinal properties.

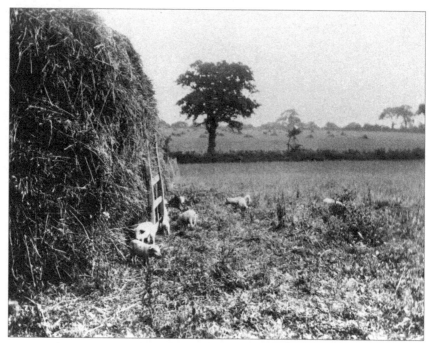

Piglets foraging around the stacks at Wood farm, Saxthorpe, in the 1930s. (© Norfolk Rural Life Museum)

1

Plant Medicine in Britain

Domestic plant medicine represents the home survival kit. Built up over the centuries, through the daily life of ordinary country people, it has been preserved with remarkable accuracy from one generation to the next. Many human discoveries about the natural world are remarkable. The knowledge of plant medicines must rank as one of the most important in terms of survival of the species. How was this knowledge gained? Was it all empirical, or did our forebears possess a greater instinctive knowledge of food and medicines, akin to that still seen in animals? Horses and cattle will seek out particular plants to eat when they are ill; domestic dogs eat grass to make themselves sick when they have stomach problems. Arthur Stanley Broome, recalling his working days in Norfolk, tells us:

On Saturday mornings in the springtime, I have been in charge of a flock of ewes and lambs grazing the roadside banks and fences. The herbs the ewes ate were considered a great benefit to their health and of medical benefit too to help them get over lambing quickly.[1]

One elderly Norfolk man who was a shepherd all his working days told me how sheep normally avoid eating ivy (*Hedera helix*) leaves, but will seek these out if they are ill. If there was no ivy available in their field, he would offer them a bunch: 'If a sheep won't eat ivy, you may as well cut its throat.'[2]

Ewart Evans reported the observation of a Suffolk horseman that horses seek out the bark of certain trees when they are ill: 'They whoolly liked to eat some trees. I'd watch 'em going to the hedge and see what trees they'd stop at. Some of my horses used to strip the bark off an oak and some would take to the ellum. Chance times I used to give 'em some of the bark grated up in their bait. It used to make their coats shine like satin.'[3] A Norfolk countryman observed that, 'if a bed of nettles in the corner of a meadow were mown and left lying for twenty-four hours, horses would eat the nettles eagerly, and benefit from them as from a tonic medicine.'[4] Recent work in Dorset suggests that Amazonian woolly monkeys, even in captivity, seek out the most appropriate herbs from those available to treat their own ailments.[5]

Many people are familiar with the spring-time craving for fresh fruit and salad, which in physiological terms makes good sense; during a long winter, it is easy to become short of vitamin C. Possibly the strange food cravings experienced by many women during pregnancy fall into the category of vestiges of an earlier more strongly developed knowledge of the food and tonic value of plants. Such knowledge was handed down orally from one generation to the next, to become part of that precious commodity, common sense. Plant remedies were modified and 'honed' by experience: they had to be accurately remembered and passed on, since otherwise toxic plants, or toxic parts of plants, could have been used with very serious effects. In the eighteenth-century records of the Presbytery of Peebles there is an account of a murder case brought before the Kirk session. Isobel F. was accused of murdering her husband, by doctoring his ale:

> She denied everything, except that she sent to the gardener's wife at Linton for some herbs, viz. Badmonnie (*Meum athamanticum*) and fumitory (*Fumaria* sp.) and thereafter implored her aunt, Mary F., to go to Ingistone for the herbs or any other place where she may get them, and that she brought them from Dolphinton. But she had no bad dealing in seeking them, but was advised that they were proper for her condition' [she was pregnant]. Will Gray his wife said that Isobel sent to her for badmonnie, but she said she had it not.[6]

Luckily for Isobel, the case was considered unproven.

This story illustrates the fact that there was a general awareness of the misuse as well as the use of herbs in medicine. Although it was rarely written down, even in relatively recent times, common knowledge of plant medicines must have been accurate to avoid catastrophes. An interesting example of this is provided by comfrey (*Symphytum officinale*), a plant used medicinally since the days of the ancient Greeks. In very recent times, doubt has been cast upon the safety of its use. Substances toxic to the liver have been identified in the leaves, and the popular press has made much of the dangers of this traditional plant remedy. What is of great interest is that traditionally the *root*, and not the leaves, of this plant was used in plant medicine. When I mentioned the use of a tea made from the leaves of comfrey to a Romany friend, he was scandalized that anyone would use the leaves; the root

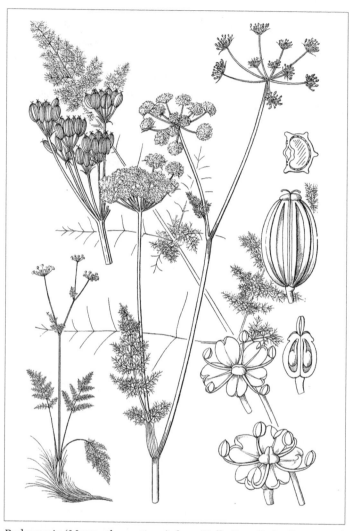

Badmonnie (*Meum athamanticum*), from Stella Ross-Craig, *Drawings of British Plants*. (By kind permission of the Royal Botanical Gardens, Kew/photograph courtesy of John Innes Foundation Historical Collections)

alone was safe to use, and this (to him) was common knowledge, far preceding in time the modern pharmacological analysis. Used in its traditional way, this remedy is perfectly safe, but modern 'secondary' use of the plant was inaccurate. The common-sense approach to plant medicine, used as part of people's everyday lives, included an awareness of which parts of a plant it was safe to use. People did not regard this as specialist information, but took it for granted as common knowledge.

For this reason, when I was collecting data on twentieth-century plant remedies, many people initially disclaimed any knowledge of the subject. If, however, I asked, 'What did your mother do for you when you were ill as a child', very often a great deal of information emerged. This is in no way a denigration of its value, more a reflection of how essential a part this knowledge played in people's lives. Clifford Geertz has defined common sense as 'a loosely connected body of belief and judgement, rather than just what anybody properly put together cannot help but think'.[7]

It is, he suggests, more than a recognition of things as they are, it involves 'how to deal with a world in which such things obtain'.[8] Before the advent of medicine as a profession in this country, a working knowledge of plant medicines was, quite literally, a vital part of this body of common sense. The great anthropologist Evans-Pritchard's description of the Azande could equally well be applied to the country people of Britain, at least up to the present century. They 'have a sound working knowledge of nature in so far as it concerns their welfare ... It is true that their knowledge is empirical and incomplete and that it is not transmitted by any systematic teaching but is handed over from one generation to another slowly and casually during childhood and early manhood, yet it suffices for their everyday tasks and seasonal pursuits.'[9]

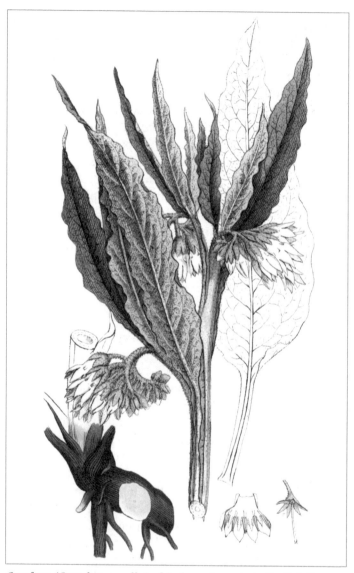

Comfrey (*Symphytum officinale*), from Sowerby's *English Botany*.
(Photograph courtesy of John Innes Foundation Historical Collections)

Knowledge of domestic medicine was handed down orally and, even after the invention of printing and the rise of literacy, very little of it was ever written down: by definition, it is knowledge used by the least literate. Yet oral testimony can be remarkably accurate, sometimes more so than the written word, which is subject to copyists' errors, misinterpretation and misrepresentation. Too often a writer has a point to make and will be selective in the information he uses to illustrate that point. Oral testimony may be highly accurate, but it rarely provides a complete picture for posterity; as the generation which used a particular knowledge dies off, so that knowledge dies too unless passed on to the next generation, or recorded in some way. I have frequently come across fragmentary knowledge of twentieth-century plant remedies; someone may remember a particular plant being used, but cannot recall how it was used; another may remember how to make a remedy, but cannot recall what it was a remedy for. This process accelerates as soon as a particular remedy is no longer in current use.

There is no motivation for the users of domestic medicine to record their remedies in writing. What few records there are on the subject have usually been written by people with no direct experience of country remedies. Such writing tends to treat fragments of information as curios, of a rather quaint nature, to be collected together like a collection of dried butterflies. This not only removes the information from its context, it also tends to lead to a condescending attitude towards the users of such remedies.

The very word 'folk' has come to have a patronizing ring to it, and too often accounts of folk medicine concentrate on the bizarre and the fanciful. Taken out of context, and sometimes even quoted quite wrongly, this has built up a picture of folk medicine as a collection of odd anachronistic rituals, practised by the ignorant and superstitious. In reality, domestic medicine was a necessary tool for survival, and still is in many countries. It represents the essence of plant wisdom of many centuries, and it is our loss if we dismiss this wisdom too lightly.

The reasons for the lack of written records of domestic medicine were simply that there was no need to write down such common knowledge, and its practitioners often could not read or write. Simply because of this, their memory was much more retentive than is ours today. It is well known that the less an ability is used, the less efficiently it functions. Today we are so used to depending on the written word that there is no strong motivation for committing large tracts of information to memory. In the past, country people were more at one with their surroundings than we are today. Many could tell the time very accurately without a watch, and predict the weather without listening to radio forecasts or recording pressure changes. The use of plants for medicine as well as for food was part of this greater attunement with the environment.

In order to remember which plant was used for which ailment, it seems likely that a system of mnemonics was developed. It was found that lesser celandine (*Ranunculus ficaria*) relieved piles; the tuberous roots look vaguely like piles, so as well as giving the name pilewort to the plant, the bumpy roots could serve as a mnemonic. This seems to me a much more convincing explanation of many of our common plant names than the so-called 'doctrine of signatures'. This famous doctrine was first proposed by Paracelsus in the sixteenth century. It is highly significant that he was himself a physician; like all the literate men of his day, he wrote at several removes from the ordinary common people and their ordinary daily life and ills. He suggested that every plant was 'marked' with its own medical use, resembling either the part of the

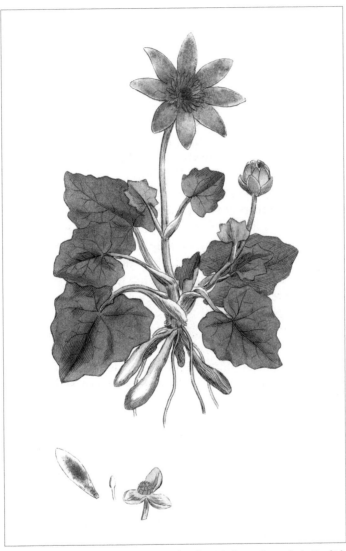

Pilewort, lesser celandine (*Ranunculus ficaria*), from Sowerby's *English Botany.* (Photograph courtesy of John Innes Foundation Historical Collections)

body to which it should be applied or the symptoms of the disease which it could cure. This so-called doctrine of signatures was expounded by various seventeenth-century English herbalists, such as William Coles and Nicholas Culpeper.[10]

Once committed to print, information takes on an authority which it does not always deserve. An anecdote from Norfolk will serve to illustrate this. Jack was born in 1900, and all his working days he led a shire horse stallion around the farms of Norfolk to serve the mares. He spent his life very largely with his horse, often sleeping alongside it in a barn. A local farmer, knowing of my interest in old remedies, had lent me an eighteenth-century book on farriery, and in this I had read that it was customary, in order to ensure that the mare fell pregnant, to beat her with a bunch of stinging nettles (*Urtica dioica*) before the stallion arrived. I was curious to know whether this practice survived into Jack's lifetime.

I felt shy and awkward with Jack, and foolish because I found it difficult to understand his very strong Norfolk accent and vocabulary. I told him of what I had read in the old book on farriery. His whole face creased up with laughter, and he laughed until the tears made runnels down his grubby face. When he had recovered sufficiently to talk, he told me, 'They books, they get it all wrong! You beat the mare *after* the stallion has been!' (which of course, in physiological terms makes a lot more sense).[11]

The doctrine of signatures may represent another prime example of a case where the books got it wrong! Might it not be the case that Paracelsus, and others following his written lead, misinterpreted an already well-established and well-used system of mnemonics, well known to the country people who actually made up and used medicines from everyday plants? The berberis (*Berberis* sp.) was not good for jaundice because it had yellow bark: its yellowness, like a jaundiced complexion, was a feature of the plant by which to remember its medical use. Once the doctrine of signatures was invented by the literate class, it became embroidered and might well have led to some misuses of plants; so that, by extension, all yellow plants might be thought good for jaundice. This idea is explored further in Chapter 5.

Domestic medicine was a common-sense collection of first aid worked out by instinct, by observation of animals and by trial and error, and, at least until the advent of printing, preserved entirely by word of mouth. With the advent of printing came an entirely new chapter in the history of plant medicine. Once committed to print, whether accurate or not, one particular remedy would be preserved and copied from one century to the next. As long as remedies were actually in use, there was little danger of their becoming inaccurate; once they fell into disuse, and particularly once they appeared as reported remedies in print, the situation became very different, and their accuracy slumped.

Any error once appearing in print has a tendency to be repeated almost indefinitely. Since the written herbals were available only to the privileged few who could read and write and afford to buy them, a divergence began between the written herbal medicine of the elite and the ordinary grassroots medicine of the majority of country people. Injected into the written record of herbal medicine was the current 'official' medical thinking of the day, as well as ideas gathered from abroad. As this process continued, herbal medicine as recorded in the literature diverged further and further from the orally transmitted traditions of country medicine. While there was occasional input from domestic medicine into 'official' medicine, there was probably very little input in the other direction, from official to traditional.

Oddly, as Oliver Wendell Holmes had pointed out, official medicine has always been strangely reluctant to acknowledge its debt to domestic medicine. As a result of this attitude, there is no doubt that much valuable information has been and continues to be lost. Yet the 'discoveries', or strictly re-discoveries, made in this way have been profoundly significant:

> It [medicine] learned from a monk how to use antimony, from a Jesuit how to cure agues, from a friar how to cut for stone, from a soldier how to treat gout, from a sailor how to keep off scurvy, from a postmaster how to sound the Eustachian tube, from a dairymaid how to prevent smallpox, and from an old market-woman how to catch the itch-insect.[12]

A striking example of an instance where domestic medicine could have helped orthodox medicine is to be found in the manuscript of the *Gunton Household Book*, a seventeenth- and eighteenth-century kitchen book kept by members of the Harbord family. Anyone who has worked with archives will know the feeling of awe and excitement they can engender. The *Gunton Household Book* is kept in the church of St Peter Mancroft, in Norwich. The first time I opened it, the sunlight was shining through the stained-glass windows on to the faded ink, and it was with a feeling of privilege that I turned the pages and familiarized myself with the handwriting of successive women of the Harbord family. For several years in the 1970s, I had worked in cancer research, and it was a moving and humbling experience to come across this early eighteenth-century remedy:

> For a sore brest yt is Painfull knotted and yet white and hard. Take flax ... and upon it ... ye herb Periwinkle, and

fume it over frankincense and apply it hot morning and evening renew it as ye herb dryes away continue this for some time and it will take ye pain quite away and disperse ye knots Prov'd by Mrs Bacon of Ipswich.[13]

Periwinkle belongs to the genus *Vinca*, which has now given its name to the vinca-alkaloids which have played such a major role in the treatment of many malignancies, and have led to the transformation in treatment of childhood leukaemia. The actual species of periwinkle used in extraction of modern vinca-alkaloids is the Madagascar periwinkle (*Vinca rosea*, now called *Catharanthus roseus*), but the common periwinkle (*Vinca minor*) has also yielded some interesting compounds currently used in treatment of arteriosclerosis and certain types of dementia. Had this group of plants come to the notice of the medical profession earlier, how many lives might have been saved?

What is the basis of the undeniable reluctance of the medical profession either to acknowledge its debt to 'popular' medicine or to take plant medicines seriously enough to investigate them thoroughly? This is a complex and interesting subject, which will be explored further in the coming chapters. Suffice it to say here that there are probably two main reasons for this reluctance. The first is a historical one: with the so-called 'rationalization' of medicine in the eighteenth century, the medical profession was at pains to distance itself from the non-scientific remedies of the past. The other major reason is a far more subtle one, and concerns the image of the medical profession, both as its practitioners wish themselves to be seen, and as their patients wish to see them.

Domestic medicine, by definition, had no distinct 'practitioners'. It was a do-it-yourself collection of first aid. However, once individuals gained reputations as

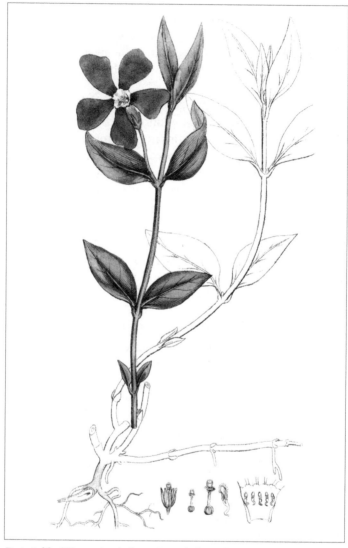

Periwinkle (*Vinca minor*), from Sowerby's *English Botany*. (Photograph courtesy of John Innes Foundation Historical Collections)

healers, they were immediately set apart from the ordinary people, and invested with special powers. We want to have faith in our healers: we want to believe that they possess greater knowledge than we do ourselves. Meanwhile the healers, set apart by their patients, will in many cases foster this image of themselves as being special, possessing extraordinary powers or knowledge. Once this happens, the healers become increasingly motivated to shroud their practice in mystery, magic, or obscure terminology. This in turn sets them still further apart from the people they treat.

Another factor in the distancing of healers from those they attempt to treat is the payment factor. In domestic medicine, money very rarely changes hands. Healers, however, have made it their job, and will expect payment in kind or in money. This presupposes that they possess knowledge not owned by those they treat; similarly, the medical professional must not be seen to be using the same old everyday remedies that everyone knows about and takes for granted. The use of Latin by the medical profession (even up to the present time) is an example of this need to emphasize that they have something special to offer, beyond the grasp of the ordinary patient. It is very difficult to find out about the healers who used plant medicine, since they kept no records. Tantalizing glimpses and stories of 'wise women' and men abound, but hard facts are difficult to come by, although there are still such healers practising in developing countries. The accounts we do have tend to confirm that, as in the case of the medical profession, once the healers are recognized as experts, they are set apart from the normal run of humanity, and their practice acquires all kinds of ritual, which is quite absent from the ordinary practice of plant medicine. Examples of this will be given in the following chapters.

This book is primarily concerned with the history of rural domestic medicine during the last three centuries, from the time when official and domestic medicine began to part company. Since, as we have seen, the practitioners of domestic plant medicine in Britain during the last three centuries were mostly ordinary, often illiterate, country people, how can we learn about the remedies that they used? Fortunately, although the medical profession was loath to recognize its common ground with the traditional users of plant medicine, such was not the case with the writers of the early herbals. In many of these herbals there are references to remedies learned from private individuals (see Chapter 2). Manuscript diaries and letters and kitchen books belonging to the seventeenth, eighteenth and nineteenth centuries are a more problematic source of information concerning the plant remedies that were actually in everyday use. Since only the wealthy landowners kept such kitchen books, it follows naturally that they reflect mainly the medicine of the well-to-do. Occasionally, however, one comes across a reference to a remedy obtained not from a fellow member of the gentry, but from a gardener, or another employee on the estate, or simply quoted as used 'by the country people'. In this way, the writings of the wealthy can offer glimpses of the domestic medicine of the ordinary people. Thus the diaries of John Clerk of Penicuik (1719–90) record remedies gleaned from the gardener, the flesher (butcher) as well as from fellow landed gentry.[14] But on the whole, kitchen books in both England and Scotland record remedies swapped from one wealthy family to another.

As home medicine and orthodox medicine diverged further during the eighteenth and nineteenth centuries, the herbalist emerged as a new alternative, and the history of herbalism is extremely well recorded by Barbara Griggs.[15] Suffice it to say here that, as a result of political manoeuvring, the English herbalists were largely forced either underground or abroad, and, as a result, many of the remedies used in British herbalism today have been re-imported from North America. As such, they represent a distillation of a quite separate tradition of plant remedies, many of them using North American rather than native British plants.

It is beyond the scope of this present book to review traditional medicine worldwide. However, much of what is said in this book about British domestic medicine could probably be applied to domestic medicine elsewhere. In general, free, local plants are used, and there is a lack of ritual and superstition surrounding them. These elements begin to creep in only when there are distinct practitioners and patients. An extreme example of this comes from a tribe in a small region of South America. Here, herbal medicine has become an exclusively male domain, so exclusive, in fact, that it is conducted, by the men alone, in a language reserved entirely for herbal medicine, and never taught to the women![16]

In general, too much has been made of the link between magic, witchcraft, superstition and plant medicine. The vast majority of British people used plant medicines as ordinary first aid. Once written down, many of the rules for using such plants became distorted. The image of the herb-gatherer only collecting plants at a certain time of the day, and in dark and shady places, has twisted the truth. It was found by experience, and is now being ratified by phytochemistry, that many plant constituents vary in their concentration, depending on the season and the growth conditions of the plant.[17] What were empirical observations have been turned by some writers into dark mysterious rituals. For example, much has been made by some folklorists of the customs of carrying acorns, conkers, or potatoes to ward off illness. I would like to suggest that such practices, like many superstitions, are vestiges of an earlier, perfectly sensible, use of the plant. Thus, in the past, remedies were made from potatoes to ease the pain of rheumatism. As the practice was discontinued, only the remnant of the remedy was remembered. Numerous other examples of such vestigial remains of remedies will be quoted in the following pages.

Our present knowledge of domestic medicine is fragmentary, much of it having been lost once the practice of it was discontinued, with few reliable written records. It is to be hoped that what remains will not be falsified further, nor recorded in too patronizing a way for posterity. In our present century, elderly people with such knowledge usually have not passed it on to the next generation, for fear of being laughed at, or simply because they feel such information is not of interest to anyone. (In the past, individuals with a wide knowledge of plant remedies had an even stronger motive for remaining silent; if they made their knowledge too obvious, they could be branded as witches.)

If a particular plant was of major importance in domestic medicine, then rules for its preservation would arise if necessary; the ban on picking certain plants, or bringing them indoors, may have arisen in this way. Every part of the elder tree has been used in plant medicine, and its importance in this area may have a bearing on its being regarded, from the time of the Druids onwards, as sacred. It is still today regarded as unlucky to cut a branch of elder; is this superstition all that is left of an earlier healthy respect for a plant that could help so many human ills? This idea is explored more fully in Chapter 3.

There is a tendency today to regard many things from the past as primitive. If primitive means closer to the natural world, then it should be used as a compliment.

Rather than dismissing items of plant lore as quaint reminders of a more ignorant past, they should be seen as clues to an earlier, far more comprehensive knowledge of the use of plants. The area of plant medicine covered in this book is mainly the history of country medicine from the beginning of the eighteenth century onwards. This was a time of dramatic change within official medicine, which became rationalized, with the loss of many formerly used simples, and began to diverge further and further from traditional plant medicine. Before this, the pharmacopoeia for both was similar, and consisted largely of native British plants. As country and official medicine diverged, the gulf between the medicine practised by rich and poor likewise enlarged. For this book, I have gathered the fragmentary evidence of the domestic practice of medicine among the rural poor. Domestic remedies did of course include all kinds of non-plant constituents, such as salt, ink, slugs and snails, urine and spittle (many of which also featured in official medicine, at least until the end of the eighteenth century). But these household remedies, however interesting their story is, are beyond the scope of this book, which deals primarily with plant remedies.

While the early origins of domestic plant medicine cannot be established with certainty, it does seem clear that such knowledge was born out of necessity. Even as recently as the eighteenth century, official medical help was inadequate and too costly to supply the needs of the rural population in Britain. Porter points out that at the beginning of the eighteenth century, Britain's roads were perhaps in a worse state than when the Romans departed![18] This was another reason why in country areas even those who could afford medical aid would be self-reliant as far as possible. As the century progressed, official medical services became more widely available, at least to those who could afford them. However, for the rural agricultural labourer, life changed little in this respect between 1700 and 1900, and even well into the twentieth century. Tom Higdon, arriving at Burston Village School as a teacher at the turn of the twentieth century, found conditions so bad for the labouring poor that he and his wife soon became instrumental in what became known as the 'Burston Rebellion'. Higdon described the conditions in poetry, but there was nothing poetic about the suffering and poverty widespread among the families of agricultural labourers:

> With tattered shoes the children trudge to school
>   Along the lanes wet slush and muddy pool, –
> Prey to diseases springing from their chills
> And to the more preventable of ills
> All for the labourer's lack of means to buy
> Clothing to keep his children warm and dry![19]

The agricultural labourer was at the bottom of the pile in terms of wage-earning, and this remained true even during the so-called golden age of agriculture in the nineteenth century. The prosperity of landowners and farmers was not shared with the labourer, whose wage remained the lowest in the national economy.[20] The basic problems of life – low income, limited food, inadequate housing – were probably similar for the agricultural labourer at the beginning of the eighteenth century to those in the early years of the twentieth century. Survival depended on hard work, luck, and self-reliance. The picture generally painted of rural England during the eighteenth century is usually of a tripartite society consisting of landowners, tenant farmers and landless wage-earners. However, as Armstrong points out, this is an oversimplification. In addition, there were small farmers, especially in the west of the country in counties such as Herefordshire, and for them living conditions may have been even harder than for the cottager. Low prices and enclosure forced many of them out of their farms, while the wealth of the large landowners increased. In the early decades of the nineteenth century, the French wars brought an increase in prices of agricultural produce, but with the advent of peace, the labour market was flooded, leading to more hardship. Average earnings for an agricultural labourer sank to a minimum in 1824.

As industry developed, there was increased migration from the countryside to the town. Overall population in both town and country increased, owing in part to a reduction in childhood mortality. As medical services, together with public health, improved in the towns and cities, rural life in many ways remained unaltered. Such medical services as were available in the country continued to be too expensive for the majority of agricultural labourers well into the twentieth century. For the rural labourer, family knowledge of domestic plant medicine must have been instrumental in keeping his animals and his family alive. By definition, there is no written record of his practice of domestic medicine: 'The labouring poor did not leave their workhouses stashed with documents for historians to work over'.[21] We therefore have to depend on fragmentary written information, and on extrapolation backwards in time from our present century. The guardians of such knowledge became fewer as the nineteenth century progressed. As Armstrong points out, the migration from countryside to town must have interrupted the transmission of country beliefs through the generations, as well as reducing the number of people who held them in common.[22]

It should be pointed out that although country medicine was a necessity for many, it was also often held in high regard, and its use was not entirely a matter of *faute de mieux*. In an eighteenth-century log book belonging to a surgeon-apothecary in Dalkeith, Scotland, he records the story of one of his patients suffering from heavy periods. He presribed for her nettles (*Urtica dioica*), 'knowing how she dislik'd all shop medicines'.[23] This lady evidently had the means necessary to consult an official practitioner, but even so she still considered the ordinary plant medicines of the countryside to be extremely valuable. Holloway is of the opinion that folk medicine 'was used more frequently and regarded more highly by the mass of the population than the advice of the medical profession'.[24]

During the nineteenth century, Poor Law medical aid and membership of the Friendly Societies became available in towns and cities, and to a lesser extent in the countryside, but it was not always seen as a preferable option. Often membership of a Friendly Society was too expensive, and in many cases covered only the named member and not his family. Even the National Insurance Scheme, introduced in 1911, provided medical cover only for the husband, for the wife if she worked, for the children not at all. The working family became 'panel patients'. The standard charge for a visit from a general practitioner to a panel patient seems to have been *2s 6d* (12.5p). The cost of medicine varied between about *6d* (2.5p) and *1s* (5p). Before the First World War, average farm wages were around *10s* (50p) to *12s* (60p) in East Anglia.[25] A quarter of a week's wages would be paid as a medical fee only in a dire emergency:

Working class people seldom saw a doctor because of the cost – a shilling to visit the surgery including medicine – if you were desperately ill the doctor came home; this cost half a crown old money. Mostly it was remedies mother had learned from her mother, or something a neighbour suggested.[26]

Given the continuing high cost of medical treatment, it is not surprising that country people retained their spirit of independence despite the advent of the Health Service. A habit of countless generations, to look after themselves for all but the most life-threatening conditions, should not be expected to vanish overnight; and indeed it did not. Perhaps this was best expressed by an old lady in Essex, speaking early in the twentieth century of the then recent birth of the National Health Service: 'we don't need all these 'ere doctors, we can look after ourself'.[27]

Even after official medical treatment did become widely available and more affordable in country areas, there were still some independent spirits who preferred to look after themselves. A locally well-known lady who inherited a farm in Norfolk in the 1930s fell off a stack when she was eighty years old, and broke both wrists. When her fellow-workers on the farm tried to persuade her to go to hospital, she retorted, 'Hospital! I haven't got time to go to hospital.' Instead, she chose to treat herslf by poulticing both wrists with comfrey from her garden, and both healed well.[28]

Nowadays there are very few people in Britain who would treat a serious medical complaint with their own plant remedies. In the past, even the relatively recent past, this was not the case. Plant remedies were the only available kind of treatment, and the rural poor could only afford the free plant remedies prepared by themselves and their families. One might expect domestic plant remedies. at least in the present century, to have been used for minor common complaints, and this is indeed the case. There are many records of remedies for coughs, colds, cuts and bruises, burns and other everyday ills, but even in these cases the severity of the condition treated would today merit hospitalization, or at very least a visit to the doctor. In Chapter 4 various examples are given of home treatment for serious injuries. On p. 250 the case is quoted of a young boy who cut the end off his thumb. This was treated by his mother, at home, with a poultice made from a lily leaf, and it healed perfectly, without a scar. An informant from Yorkshire remembers being treated by her grandfather for what was obviously a serious cut (p. 151), while a lady brought up on the edge of a forest recalls her granny treating an infected foot with great success (p. 157).

It is yet more surprising to find on record twentieth-century home remedies for conditions such as appendicitis. The following recipe was collected in the 1920s from a Suffolk branch of the Women's Institute:

> Inflammation of appendix should be treated with elder and peppermint, and a compress wrung out of the same liquor applied to the bowels. If the patient has been troubled with constipation inject into the bowels one pint of elder tea, and one of hot water: 30 minutes after inject 2 quarts of hot water, and when the bowels have been entirely cleansed, cease the injections, continue the compress, and give repeated doses of the herb until a bath of perspiration follows; keep patient one temperature for 12 hours.[29]

The same collector, Mark Taylor, recorded a number of home remedies for cancer, including a poultice made from hemlock (*Conium maculatum*), or from carrot (*Daucus carota*);[30] and one made from the narrow-leaved dock (*Rumex* sp.).[31] Cancer of the liver was apparently sometimes treated with a decoction made from celandine (presumably this was the greater celandine, *Chelidonium majus*),[32] and it was written that the poultice made from narrow-leaved dock 'has been known to cure a growth on a man's hand'.

A caveat is necessary here: it is impossible to be sure of the diagnosis in modern medical terms of a condition treated in the past. Jaundice, for example, was treated as a single complaint: nowadays it is regarded as a symptom of a number of different conditions. The same caution is necessary in interpreting remedies for cancer: skin cancers in particular are difficult to define, and obviously folk remedies would not distinguish between the benign and the so-called premalignant forms of rodent ulcers. For this reason, any apparent records of 'cures' must be interpreted with caution.

I have come across several references to the belief that 'the cure is out there'; that for every ailment, there exists a herb that will cure it. Doubtless this was a comforting belief in an age where orthodox medicine had little more to offer than did folk medicine, or indeed when medical treatment was too expensive to be generally available. It was, however, recognized that some conditions were difficult or impossible to treat. Rheumatism, for instance, was regarded as intractable. The self-styled King of the Norfolk Poachers left in his writings some vivid accounts of the herbal treatments used by his grandmother. He told us:

My grandmother had a cure of sorts for evrything, and herbs for evry complaint. The Misseltoes was a shure cure for the Hoping [whooping] Cought. Secenction[33] was a good thing for boils, Celendine for weak eys, and Plantain for Limbago, all could be cured some way or another except the rhumatics, and I think that is incurable.[34]

It would be interesting to find whether a detailed study of remedies for this complaint would reveal a greater diversity of remedies than for a more tractable condition. This is certainly the impression that East Anglian studies have given: in a recent study by the author, almost twenty plant remedies were recorded for treating rheumatic complaints in East Anglia, although wider studies are needed to confirm or refute this picture.

Obviously, the first people to experiment with herbal remedies would have used those plants near at hand: one might therefore expect the commonest plants to have been used the most in folk medicine, and this does seem to be the case. In the past, writers such as the eighteenth-century botanist Dillenius have claimed that it was a 'special providence of the Creator'[35] which determined that in any given area there were to be found plants to treat the ailments most common in that region. It would seem that, once again, learned writers might have turned the truth on its head, as with the doctrine of signatures. It is probable that early settlers anywhere would use the local plants to treat their ailments: indeed, the local flora was the only Materia Medica available to the majority. It seems much more likely that the commonness of a plant dictated its frequency of use for local ailments, rather than it corresponding to ailments specific to that locality. In this respect, the work of D.E. Allen is beginning to provide evidence for the geographical distribution of folk remedies in Britain.[36] His research tends to confirm a regional variation in the use of plant remedies which at least in some cases mirrors the distribution of those particular plants.

Some common plants, widely distributed throughout Britain, have been used for a very wide variety of ailments. This prompted one informant to write: 'Nettle tea we had to drink to purify our blood, Grandpa (unwillingly) for his sciatica and Aunt Rose for her pleurisy. I wondered how it knew which it was supposed

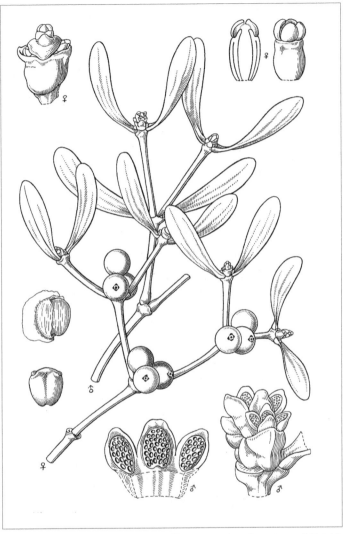

Mistletoe (*Viscum album*), from Stella Ross-Craig, *Drawings of British Plants.* (By kind permission of the Royal Botanical Gardens, Kew/ photograph courtesy of John Innes Foundation Historical Collections)

to do.'[37] Knowing as we do now the enormous number of possible 'active' compounds within one plant, multiple uses of a single plant should not come as a surprise. One species could indeed provide a whole pharmacopoeia. It is only our present single-drug medicine that has changed our way of thinking, so that we imagine that a single compound must be responsible for the effectiveness of a plant remedy. The attempt to isolate a single active principle from a plant is often doomed to failure, and can result in rejection by orthodox medicine of a perfectly effective remedy. Clearly the parameters needed to judge the effects of whole plant extracts must be different from those used to assess a single known compound. Increasingly, it is being shown that the effect of a whole plant extract is different from that of a known active principle within it. The phenomenon of 'synergism', where the effect of the sum of plant compounds is different from their separate effects, is also being recognized. For these reasons, it would be unwise to reject as medically inactive plant remedies which have been used in folk medicine for a wide variety of ailments.

The concept of 'tonics' is an interesting one in this connection. It seems that right up to the twentieth century, the value of spring tonics was recognized. Nettle beer, dandelion (*Taraxacum officinale*) and burdock (*Arctium lappa*) beer, goosegrass (*Galium aparine*) and nettle, are all examples of homemade drinks that were regarded as pick-me-ups after the winter. A woman born in 1917 recalls: 'Great emphasis was placed on keeping the bowels open and the pores closed and of cleansing the blood after the rigours of winter and so, in the spring, we were sent to gather young nettles.'[38] Sometimes a spring pudding was made, for example in Norfolk nettle pudding was made from white of egg and steamed nettles.[39] Although a precise definition was not given for their value, such tonics were generally regarded as a boost to health after the winter. Since many plants contain vitamin C, at the very least these tonics might have made up for a winter diet deficient in fruit and vegetables.

Looking at the range of ailments treated with domestic remedies, some conditions are conspicuous by their absence. Perhaps the most notable are gynaecological complaints and contraception. Does this mean that these conditions were not treated with domestic medicine? It seems more likely that reticence concerning these matters explains the lack of records. Even in the twentieth century, such matters were not freely discussed. When informants were questioned directly about period pain, for example, little information was forthcoming. This may be due to greater stoicism in the past, or, probably, it simply reflects a shyness about discussing such things.

Naturally, there was less inhibition in talking in general terms about what 'people' used, rather than at a personal level. One lady reported that tansy (*Tanacetum vulgare*) was used for painful periods.[40] Another informant wrote of the mugwort (*Artemisia vulgaris*) which his father grew in their garden for the 'irregularities peculiar to women'.[41] An interesting letter from County Mayo, Ireland, records the use of houseleek (*Sempervivum tectorum*) as an abortifacient. The writer of the letter was told by an elderly neighbour:

It's a strange plant, that! Now, if a young girl got into 'trouble', her mother would take some of those plants, boil them and give the water to her daughter to drink. Later on she would tell the girl to climb up on a high wall and jump down. That would make the girl all right.

When, a few years ago, I related this story to a young farmer of this locality, he answered: 'It's quite true. I saw these plants tested only a short time ago. Walter C——

came to me and asked me if I had anything to give his cow that had retained the "cleansing" (afterbirth) after calving. I made up a bottle for him with *buachaill a' tighe*. Walter took it home and gave it to his cow. A few hours later she passed the "cleansing" and was all right.'

Buachaill a' tighe is one of several names that Irish has for *Sempervivum tectorum*. I should translate it as 'The Warden of the House'.[42]

In general, first-hand information on this subject is sparse, although Nurse Sheldon, a district nurse in Yorkshire in the 1950s, gave some remarkable evidence concerning home remedies and contributed a large number of such remedies to the English Folklore Survey at that time. Perhaps because she was a nurse, she had no hesitation in writing about the sensitive subjects of abortion and contraception. For 'difficult monthlies or menstruation' she records that 'peppermint with poppy seeds scalded is given'. She also cites the use of pennyroyal (*Mentha pulegium*), 'to get a woman to abort if she has too many children'. Significantly, it was given with Holland's Gin, at the time of a period, every time: assuming the pennyroyal worked, the woman would therefore not know whether or not she had been pregnant. This would make the method more acceptable to many.

Pennyroyal (*Mentha pulegium*) has had a long history as an abortifacient, and is still sometimes (unofficially) used for this purpose; even now, when abortion is more readily available, many people would prefer to quietly sort the matter out themselves. The following extract from an essay written for Age Concern, Essex, vividly paints a picture of a time in the early decades of the twentieth century when life was very hard and another pregnancy could be the last straw for a woman. It was contributed by

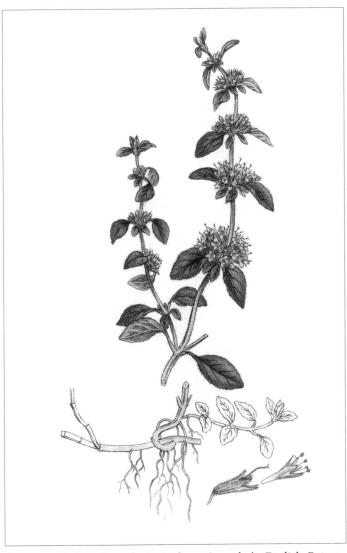

Pennyroyal (*Mentha pulegium*), from Sowerby's *English Botany*. (Photograph courtesy of John Innes Foundation Historical Collections)

four elderly women and compiled by two staff members at a day centre:

> Many of these simple stories evoked painful memories. Some of these concerned the women's knowledge, or lack of it, surrounding contraception, and when that failed, abortion. As naive young girls they were frightened into celibacy with tales of the rejection that would follow if they 'got into trouble'. Rather than being informed, they were misled with tales of how cuddling would lead directly to pregnancy; even so, as girls, they had envisaged that a little more was involved in the creation of a child. Once married and their reputations safe, the women turned to more practical methods of avoiding unwanted pregnancies. One barrier method involved soaking a sponge in vinegar; it would seem that a considerable amount of human progress owes itself to this simple condiment.
>
> Married or single, should unwanted conception take place, physical exercise was often the first option. The women would be urged to walk, big strides were best, jump down stairs, stretch and lift heavy objects. For sale were compounds such as Widow Welsh's Female Pills and Pennyroyal, said to work only in the early stages of pregnancy. We got the impression that taking this course of action was seen as a necessary evil, becoming a form of birth control in itself. Premature labour was also hoped for by drinking gin (for its juniper oil) and slippery elm. It would seem that these remedies often failed and more mechanical means were sought. When recalling the risks of illness and death surrounding back street abortions, the staff were drawn back into social circumstances which were outside their experience.[43]

Juniper (*Juniperus* spp.), as well as pennyroyal (*Mentha pulegium*), has a reputation for use as an abortifacient. As

Juniper oil was a component of gin this would explain the widespread use of gin, even in recent times, when attempting to end unwanted pregnancies. Slippery elm (*Ulmus fulva*), the other herb reputed to be an abortifacient, is a North American plant normally used for healing coughs and skin inflammation, and as an enema for constipation. It must have been bought from the chemist, since it does not grow here: clearly this is not strictly a British folk remedy.

Nurse Sheldon also mentions that if a woman was unfaithful to her husband herbagrass (herb of grace) was given to her 'to reduce her activity of ova'. Herb of grace is rue (*Ruta graveolens*). Interestingly, this is one of the plants noted by Riddle for its widespread and persistent use in contraception.[44] Nurse Sheldon further states that 'Rue tea is given to sons, and male members of the household, with same effect, to cure "Jealousy".'[45] I have been unable to trace any plant remedies specifically used for contraception. Riddle, among others, has suggested that many so-called 'emmenagogues', that is to say plants which brought on periods, were in fact used as contraceptives, and that early abortion was perhaps one of the main methods of contraception. Certainly, the quotation from Essex (p. 52) suggests that this was sometimes the case. Riddle's work has caused controversy, particularly the claims that he makes for the effectiveness of home remedies in limiting population growth. However, there can be little doubt that our forebears did know about plants that caused early abortion, and therefore it is reasonable to suppose these were used in limiting family size.

Working in East Anglia in the 1920s, Mark Taylor recorded the following plants as being used to procure abortions: savin (*Juniperus* sp.) put into the teapot with ordinary tea, pennyroyal given in fairly large doses, and saffron (*Crocus sativus*) given as tea. He also recorded the use of 'heira peika or hikey pikey'. This last is presumably hiera picra, an official preparation used as a purgative. Buchan, in his eighteenth-century book *Domestic Medicine*, gives the recipe for this. It was composed of succotrine aloes (*Aloe* sp.), Virginian snakeroot (*Aristolochia serpentaria*) and ginger (*Zingiber officinalis*), infused in mountain wine and brandy.[46] Clearly here we are getting out of the realm of homely self-medication; these ingredients are none of them native plants, and such preparations would be costly. However, this in itself is of interest. It seems that in the realm of contraception and abortion there probably were no sure-fire home remedies, and women, if sufficiently desperate, would have recourse to expensive medication, perhaps in preference to mechanical abortion. In her book *Victorian Women*, Joan Perkin refers to a woman in Dudley in the early years of the twentieth century who aborted after taking 'Hickey-Pickey, bitter aloes, white diachylon – one pennyworth of each'.[47] Diachylon, still included in the *British Pharmaceutical Codex* for 1923, is prepared from lead and olive oil, and was officially used as a soothing agent for eczema and other skin conditions. It could therefore be bought at a chemist shop. Hickey-pickey (hiera picra), as we have seen, was originally composed of aloes, snakeroot and ginger. Virginian snakeroot (*Aristolochia serpentaria*) is a North American plant known, along with other related species, as 'birthwort', and used, from the time of Dioscorides, to ease labour. Its use as an abortifacient was doubtless unofficial. A present-day herbalist describes birthwort as 'a very dangerous abortifacient'.[48] But this, too, would have been available at a chemist shop, since it was included in the *British Pharmaceutical Codex*, where its use is given as a bitter for treatment of dyspepsia.[49] Even hiera picra still appears in the 1923 *British Pharmaceutical Codex*, but, significantly, its components are listed simply as aloes and cinnamon.

How widespread was the use of birthwort as an abortifacient? This is impossible to answer. It is of interest to note that birthwort was grown in abbey gardens, and indeed was still present in large quantities, naturalized, in the garden of Carrow Abbey in Norwich as recently as 1968.[50] Carrow Abbey was once a Benedictine nunnery, where doubtless the plant was grown for its medicinal use in easing labour in those they treated, and perhaps (unofficially) in aiding abortion.

Abortion seems to have been one area where even the poor country-dweller might have to pay for treatment. The following extract from Mary Webb's novel, *The Golden Arrow*, suggests the fear and secrecy that inevitably accompanied an effort to procure abortion. The pregnant heroine is considering a visit to Nancy, a woman known for her herbal cures:

> Her acknowledged patients ... she prescribed for with surprising efficiency; her cures were simple, often drastic, usually very sensible. But her real patients – those who made her income – came in the evening, closely shrouded. They crept up to her shut door and curtained window through the colewort and butterbur at the foot of the gaunt mounds.[51]

This book of course is fiction, but is based on the author's experience of life in Shropshire. That such women as Nancy really existed, there can be little doubt, and the overlap between the role of midwife and healer is discussed in Chapter 4. It seems highly likely that such individuals were also called upon to help procure abortions, although naturally no records would be kept, and so we will probably never know how common this was.

Riddle records his own surprise at the evidence for an unwritten knowledge among country women concerning abortion and contraception.[52] Yet all over the world, such knowledge as there was would probably have been passed on from mother to daughter. Given the secrecy surrounding the whole subject of human reproduction, and the sensitivity of the issue of abortion in particular, it is not surprising that we have no more than glimpses of the use of plants in this area. Once, when giving a talk to a small local village meeting, I asked for information about the uses of one particular common plant. An elderly man told me that he knew of a use for it, but he couldn't possibly tell me. When pressed, he still did not want to tell me. After the meeting, I asked whether he could tell me privately what this use was, and he did so, in a whisper. The plant (*Galium aparine*) was fed to stallions in the spring to increase their seed. If this much shyness surrounded animal reproduction, how much less willing must people have been to talk about abortion in human beings!

It is possible that there are hidden clues to be found in popular poetry and sayings. For example, although gorse (*Ulex europaeus*) flowers all year round, there is a proverb that 'Love is out of fashion when the gorse is out of bloom'. Gorse flowers were used in Suffolk as an emmenagogue (provoking periods).[53] Were they perhaps also used as a contraceptive, available all the year round?

This East Anglian ballad about thyme (*Thymus vulgaris*) and rue (*Ruta graveolens*) may well have a double meaning:

> Come all young women and maids
> That are all in your prime

Mind how you plant your gardens gay
Let no one steal your thyme

Once I had thyme enough
To last me night and day
There came to me a false young man
Stole all my thyme away

And now my thyme is done
I cannot plant no new,
There lays the bed where my old thyme grew,
't's all over-run with rue.

Rue is running root
Runs all across amain
If I could pluck that running root
I'd plant my old thyme again.[54]

This ballad could be taken at its face value. However, thyme was known as an emmenagogue.[55] It might perhaps have been used as an abortifacient, and this may be the implication of the ballad. Rue, likewise, was used as an emmenagogue. Riddle suggests that the giving of a pot of rue to a daughter on her wedding day, a custom that persists in modern Lithuania, is a similar vestige of its former use.[56] In the areas of contraception and abortion, even more than in other areas of health, it is extremely difficult to find out about the practice of domestic medicine.

These examples serve to illustrate the fragmentary knowledge of domestic plant medicine that has survived into present times. Given that, like so much of rural life, it is part of an essentially oral tradition, we should be grateful that even this much has survived. The British were a greener nation in the past, with a built-in

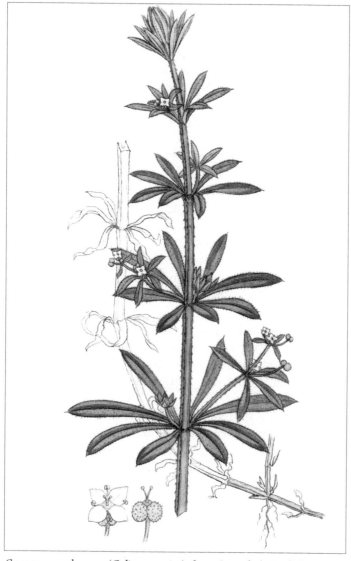

Goosegrass, cleavers (*Galium aparine*), from Sowerby's *English Botany*. (Photograph courtesy of John Innes Foundation Historical Collections)

knowledge of plant medicines that is now largely lost. Domestic medicine in this country during the last three hundred years was a common-sense aid to daily survival, not a quaint collection of bizarre practices. This book is an attempt to set the record straight, as well as to record for posterity some of the remaining fragments of knowledge of this country medicine so well known to our forebears.

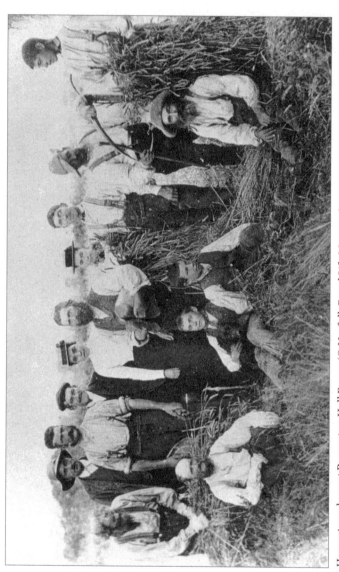

Harvest workers at Brampton Hall Farm. (© Norfolk Rural Life Museum)

2

WHAT DO WE KNOW ABOUT COUNTRY REMEDIES?

There are several sources of information concerning domestic plant remedies used during the last three hundred years in Britain. The first is written material, both manuscript and printed. The second is poetry and proverbs. The third is evidence from the names given to the plants used. The fourth is oral testimony of those who have used these remedies within living memory. Each of these major sources will be discussed in turn.

I. Written Sources

By definition, domestic medicine is primarily a practical system of first-aid measures, employed in the past by people who could not afford orthodox medical treatment. Its practitioners were ordinary people, often illiterate, and unlikely to keep records of any of their day-to-day activities. An exception to this is the kitchen books kept by the heads of wealthy households: these manuscripts include a few 'traditional' plant remedies alongside advice from the orthodox medical profession, and from printed books of the day. Can they also provide some insight into the remedies used by the mass of people? In some cases, they certainly can. The source of information is sometimes given, as in the examples below, taken from eighteenth- and nineteenth-century manuscripts.

Among the Clerk of Penicuik family papers[1] there are numerous remedies for 'The Gravell', collected by successive generations of the family who suffered from this painful complaint (kidney stones). In the latter part of the seventeenth century, John Clerk wrote down a collection of these, including remedies collected from the Laird of Innes, Lady Roslin, Lady Crimont, 'John Tarts wife who dwells in Prestoun-pans' and 'David Livingstoun, wheelwright, Dalkeith'. Presumably, these latter two remedies may represent a fragment of traditional domestic medicine: they are unlikely to originate from orthodox medical advice; a wheelwright in seventeenth-century Scotland probably could not afford the services of a doctor. Unfortunately the remedy provided by John Tart's wife is indecipherable. David Livingstoun recommended grated carrot in white wine. The provenance of remedies collected from fellow aristocrats is difficult to establish: they could be from orthodox medical sources, or from printed books of the day, or they could themselves be family remedies.

Was domestic medicine really different for the rich and the poor? Certainly many of the remedies recorded in kitchen books and other manuscript sources include costly ingredients, which a labourer could not afford. But were these elaborate remedies actually used, even by those who could afford them? In some cases there are internal clues in the manuscript sources. For example, in the eighteenth-century *Gunton Household Book*,[2] written by successive generations of the Harbord family, there are numerous remedies for a single complaint. Some of these are recognizable from the orthodox practice of the day, or from printed sources such as magazines and newspapers, some are evidently prescriptions (the Harbord family had as a friend and family physician the famous Sir Thomas Browne) and others have been copied from printed books. These remedies have all been carefully recorded, but is there any way of knowing which of them were actually used? Occasionally there may be a comment regarding their effectiveness, or otherwise. On the envelope containing a collection of remedies for gravel in the Clerk of Penicuik papers, there is a poignant note written by a later member of the family: 'I am afraid this disease may be hereditary ... I now at the age of 46 begin to feel it ... and must prepare a stock of patience suitable to so tormenting a disease.' The note is dated 20 April 1722. It would be fascinating to know whether this member of the family tried all the remedies listed by his forebears, and if he did, whether any of them brought any relief.

Occasionally in a manuscript there is positive evidence of a remedy being used, as in a receipt for headache among the early eighteenth-century Broughton Cally papers.[3] The remedy consists of seeds and syrup of 'nymphae' (presumably *Nymphaea*, water lily), as an emulsion in water 'which my son use in france'. Sir John Clerk kept a diary largely about his own state of health, and gives the following recommendation for smoking coltsfoot (*Tussilago farfara*):

I am constantly use to smock it mixt with Tobacco not for any internal malady, but to weaken my Tobacco which otherways I find affects my head with dulness and likewise my nerves.

The Herb is commonly called Colts-foot from the shape of it, it is green above and something whiteish below and is

found in plenty on sides of rivers and amongst the sand
and gravel and in the garden of Mavisbank.

I dri it in the sun or at a fire and after removing the
Husks of it I cut it small like Tobacco for smoking In
mixing it I take equal quantities of Tobacco not by weight
but as near as I can guess by little Heaps.

There is a further note as follows: 'N.B. 30 June 1749
after a years trial I think I have benefite by it for I have less
cough than formerly tho in the 73 year of my Age'. Then
three years later, he writes, 'Note 5 August 1752 After
several years experience I have found nothing better for
an inveterate Cogh and cold than smoaking of Tusselago
as above.'[4] Sir John Clerk evidently learnt this remedy
directly from his reading of Pliny's *Natural History*, which
he quotes and translates at the beginning of the remedy.

Two and a half centuries later, I was chatting to a
gardener in Lanarkshire, when he was doubled up with a
paroxysm of coughing. 'I need my dishyluggs!' he gasped.
When he realized that I didn't know what dishyluggs was,
he led me to a patch of the garden where coltsfoot was
growing wild. 'That's dishyluggs' he explained, clearly
incredulous that anyone could not know this. It was then
that I understood the name 'dishyluggs' was presumably a
corruption of *Tussilago*, the botanical name for coltsfoot.
Again, in the 1980s, I was to hear how dried coltsfoot was
rolled into cigarettes by farm labourers in Salhouse,
Norfolk, during the Second World War. This was from
necessity, rather than as a remedy, but maybe it helped
their smoker's cough too! The coltsfoot story illustrates
several important points, including the overlap between
written and oral sources of information concerning plant
remedies. Neither the Lanarkshire gardener nor the
Salhouse farm labourer would have read Pliny: yet like the
more erudite Sir John, they used coltsfoot as tobacco.

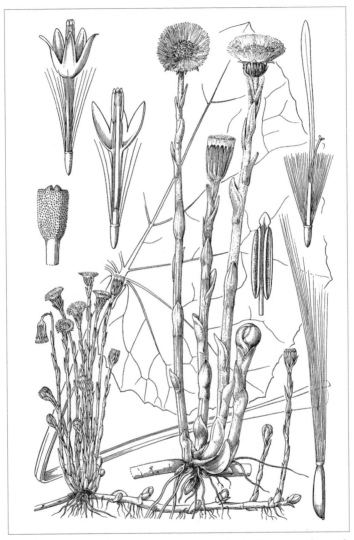

Coltsfoot (*Tussilago farfara*), from Stella Ross-Craig, *Drawings of British Plants*. (By kind permission of the Royal Botanical Gardens, Kew/ photograph courtesy of John Innes Foundation Historical Collections)

Their source of the information would presumably have been oral tradition. What was Pliny's source? Presumably oral tradition!

Such direct evidence of usage is unusual; however, there are sometimes small details given concerning the preparation of a remedy that definitely *suggest* it was a used, rather than simply a recorded, remedy. A modern analogy would be to look at someone's collection of cookery books; the well-thumbed and annotated recipes are likely to be the ones actually tried and tested. In the *Gunton Household Book* there are several remedies, among the many hundreds recorded, which would appear to have been actually used. Here is an example. After describing an ointment to 'take away wens', composed of butter, broom flowers (*Cytisus scoparius*) and elder flowers (*Sambucus nigra*), the writer adds, 'I have known it rot away a wen which was biger than a half penny Loaf'.

There are sometimes details given in a recipe that suggest that the writer has actually prepared it, as in this remedy for jaundice, also in the *Gunton Household Book*: 'Take Strawberry roots leaves and Red Strings altogether as they grow, wash them and boyle them in reasonable strong beer very well, and give ye patient to drink morning and evening a good draught'. Occasionally, testimony as to the effectiveness of a remedy is included, as in the following two examples.

A remedy for black jaundice consisting of powdered saffron (*Crocus sativus*) drunk in white wine 'was proved upon a man at Darsham that made black water as black as Ink'. A remarkable remedy for a sore breast was, we are told, 'prov'd by Mrs Bacon of Ipswich' (Chapter 1, p. 32). Powdered saffron and honey, for eyes that are extremely inflamed, 'cured severall whose eyes were almost covered with red'.[5] A more recent manuscript from Norfolk is the diary of Maryanne Weston of Thorpe. This includes various home remedies, including the following for a scurfy head in a child:

To cure the coming off of childrens hair attended with a dry humour, and scurfiness. Slightly bruise the full green but tender leaves of House leek, strain the juice and add to it a little cream. Moisten a piece of soft old Irish linnen several times double with it, till wet through, put it on the affected part when the child goes to bed at night keeping it as moist as you can all night and wash it well off in the morning with soft soap and water.

This I found a perfect cure – E.A.W.[6]

Although the majority of manuscript kitchen books contain elaborate and costly remedies, which may or may not have been used in practice, a notable exception is the fascinating page of notes on herbal remedies from the papers of the Carleton family of Norwich. There is no date on this page, but the collection of papers with which they occur covers the period 1772–c.1914. What is interesting about these particular notes is that they read like memos to the writer, and consist, not of elaborate remedies, but of simples. Here is a sample:

Radishes (*Raphanus sativus*) eaten are not very good they releive the urin much The seed of Rocket (*Sisymbrium* sp.) is used to cure the Bite of Mad Dogs and it serves to help digestion

Winter Rocket or Cresses (*Rorippa* spp.) good for ulcers Sores and ... the juice drank inwardly or applied outwardly dry and heal

The Hips of the Wild Bryer (*Rosa canina*) when quite ripe made into a syrup is good for binding the Bowells

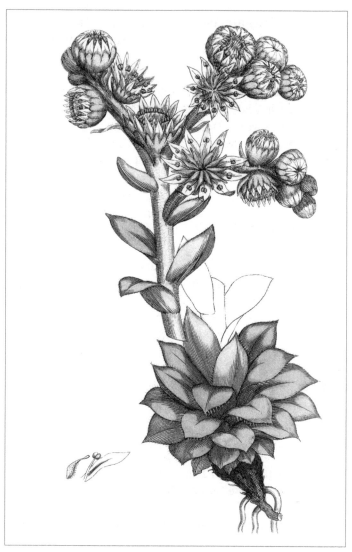

Houseleek (*Sempervivum tectorum*), from Sowerby's *English Botany*.
(Photograph courtesy of John Innes Foundation Historical Collections)

Sanicle (*Sanicula europaea*) the Roots and leaves Boild and taken is Good for many Inward Complaints sweeten with sugar

a Drink made from the Shepheards Purse (*Capsella bursa-pastoris*) is good for my complaint Ointment of the same is good for Wounds.[7]

At a guess, the writer is a woman, and 'her complaint' was presumably a gynaecological one, such as heavy periods (for which shepherd's purse is still used today), about which she was too shy to write even in her personal papers.

Even veterinary manuscripts sometimes provide information about human remedies. The following examples are taken from the eighteenth-century Kingsbury notebook, which consists mainly of remedies for horses and cows:

For the yellow jaunders in a Cristain Take Burdock (*Arctium lappa*) root Clean it and Scrap it as you would horse Radish and make it into tea and Drink it as often as you Please or till you are Cured

For weak Eyes such as Inflamation in A Cristain take watter Cresses and pulverise them in a mortar then Squeeze them close and dress your eyes with the Same

For a Liver Complaint in a Cristain Elecompana (*Inula helenium*) root, Liqurice (*Glycyrrhiza glabra*), sugar and beer

For a Complaint in the Liver in a Cristain take a good handful of DandyLion (*Taraxacum officinale*) and boil it down pretty well then sweeten it to your own taste and take a tea cup full of it 2 or 3 times a day as you think proper

These remedies sound distinctly preferable to some of those listed for horses and cows. The use of 'Elecompana' is of particular interest. Elecampane (botanical name

Inula helenium) is a herb much used by horsemen right up to the twentieth century. Ewart Evans mentions its use in restoring the appetite of a tired horse.[8] Huntingfield Women's Institute recorded its use in the 1920s for treating coughs (in humans): 'Elicampaign roots dried and grated in a spoonful of sugar'.[9] A few of the remedies in the Kingsbury notebook are considered suitable for man or beast: 'For the gravell in Horse or Cristain, Oil of Juniper one 1/4 of oz, sweet spirits of Nitre 1/2 an oz, Laudenham One Drahm, give a Horse an Oz, and a Cristain a Small tea spoon full in warm beer'.[10]

It would be natural for horsemen to try out some of the remedies on themselves, especially if they could obtain them free. In much more recent times, 'horse oils' were frequently used in East Anglia as a rub for rheumatism.[11] The area of animal remedies and its overlap with human ones is a fascinating one, made more difficult by the secrecy that often surrounded animal remedies. Many horsemen would burn their notebooks rather than pass on the information to another. I have spoken to one man whose father did just this; he refused to divulge his remedies to his son because the latter was not intending to be a horseman;[12] instead he made a bonfire of them!

> It was a well known fact that many a good old horseman has taken to his grave in animal treatment, what others would like to know about but never did. They are now recognised as concoctions but those treatments somehow worked well and it was a very rare case to see a veterinary on the farm.[13]

Sometimes even the wealthy appeared to choose home medication. This is from a letter written in 1699 by Christian Kilpatrick to her husband, Sir John Clerk:

Jamie has taken the smallpox ... I have sent in Sandy for some saffron and marigold (*Calendula officinalis*) for I have none. I give him marigold posset to drink ... I will give him some saffron inwardly when it comes, in a spoonful of claret wine and bind some of it about his throat to prevent the soreness at it.[14]

This method of treatment sounds preferable to the heroic and polypharmaceutical treatment recommended by the famous Dr Archibald Pitcairne, and recorded in 1704 among the Clerk of Penicuik papers. It includes blistering plasters and an emulsion consisting of a vast number of ingredients.[15]

To the extent that manuscripts provide examples of home remedies that were actually used, these are valuable sources of information concerning domestic plant medicine. Even printed sources can provide crumbs of information. Sometimes the authors of herbals relate anecdotes of remedies mentioned in their books. Here are some examples from John Pechey's *Compleat Herbal* of 1694:

The water of Arsmart [*Polygonum hydropiper*] is of great use in the Stone ... A Country Gentleman us'd a Load of this Herb in a Year to make the Water, wherewith he cured many of the Stone.[16]

Country-people cure Wounds with Brook-lime [*Veronica beccabunga*], mix'd with a little Salt, and a Spider's Web, and applied to the Wound, wrapp'd about with a double Cloth[17]

A Person that had the Stone, and had tried many Medicines to no purpose, was wonderfully releiv'd by the following Remedy. *I took*, says he, *two handfuls of the Flowers of the Common Camomile* [*Chamaemelum nobile*],

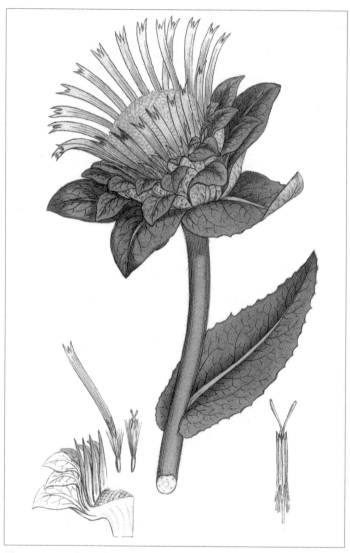

Elecampane, horseheal (*Inula helenium*), from Sowerby's *English Botany*. (Photograph courtesy of John Innes Foundation Historical Collections)

which I infus'd in a quart of Rhenish-Wine ... I took two or three Spoonfuls ... some Stones came away by Urine, without any great pain. Afterwards I prescrib'd the same for several Others that were so afflicted, who found also much Relief.[18]

The Country-people in the West of *England* use the herb (Cudweed [*Filago vulgaris*]) infus'd in Oyl, to take off Black and Blue of Bruises and Stripes.[19]

The Women in *Suffolk* boyl it (Dittander [*Lepidium latifolium*]) in Beer, to facilitate Delivery.

Shepherd's-Purse ... 'tis outwardly used by the Common People, to heal Wounds, with good success.[20]

Another example of a traditional plant remedy that eventually appeared in print is the use of mallow (*Malva* sp.) for treating wounds. The *Modern Farrier* by A. Lawson was published in London in 1842. The author quotes from Mr W. Cobbett ('none will deny his ability as a writer, and his skill as a farmer'):[21]

I cannot help mentioning here another herb which is used for medical purposes. I mean the wild mallows. It is a weed that has leaves somewhat like a scallop. Its branches spread upon the ground. It bears seed which the children call cheeses, and which they string upon a thread like beads. This weed is perhaps amongst the most valuable of plants that ever grew. Its leaves stewed, and applied wet, will cure, and almost instantly cure, any cut or bruise or wound of any sort. Poultices made of it will cure sprains, as those of the ancle: fomenting with it will remove swellings. Applications of the liquor will cure the wringings by saddles and harness. And its operation is in all cases so quick that it is hardly to be believed. Those who

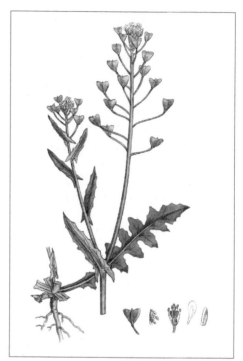

Shepherd's purse (*Capsella bursa-pastoris*), from Sowerby's *English Botany*. (Photograph courtesy of John Innes Foundation Historical Collections)

have this weed at hand need not put themselves to the trouble and expense of sending to doctors and farriers upon trifling occasions. It signifies not whether the wound be old or new. I gained this piece of information upon Long Island, from a French gentleman who was one of Bonaparte's followers in captivity, and who was afterwards robbed of three hundred dollars on board an English frigate, never having been able to obtain either remuneration or redress. The hospitality shown him by me was amply repaid by this piece of knowledge. The mallows, if you have it growing near you, may be used directly after it is gathered, merely washing off the dirt first. But there should be some always in the house ready for use. It should be gathered like other herbs, just before it comes out in bloom, and dried and preserved just in the same manner as other herbs. It should be observed, however, that if it should happen not to be gathered at the best season, it may be gathered at any time. I made a provision of it in the month of October, long after the bloom and even the seed had dropped off. The root is pretty nearly as efficacious as the branches; and it may be preserved and dried in the same manner. We all know what plague and what expence attend the getting of tinctures and salves, some of which very often prove injurious rather than otherwise. I had two striking instances of the efficacy of the mallows. A neighbouring farmer had cut his thumb in a very dangerous manner, and, after a great deal of doctoring, it was got to such a pitch that his hand was swelled to twice its natural size. I recommended the use of mallows to him: gave him a little bunch out of my store, it being winter time, and his hand was well in four days. He could go out to his work the very next day, after having applied the mallows overnight. The other instance was this: I had a pig: indeed it was a large and valuable hog, that had been gored by the sharp horn of a cow. It had been in this state two days before I knew of the accident, and had eaten nothing. My men had given it up for lost. I had the hog caught and held down. The gore was in the side, and so large and deep that I could run my finger in beyond the ribs. I poured in the liquor in which the mallows had been stewed, and rubbed the side well with it besides. The next day the hog got up and began to eat. I had him caught again; but, upon examining the wound I found it so far closed up that I did not think it right to disturb it. I bathed the side over again; and in two days, the hog was turned out, and running about along with the rest. Now, a person must be almost criminally careless not to make provision of this herb. Mine was nearly two years' old when I made use of it upon the last mentioned occasion. It is found every where, by the sides of the highway, and therefore may be come at and possessed without either trouble or expence. A good handful ought to be well boiled and stewed in about a pint of water, till it comes perhaps to half a pint. It surely is worthwhile, especially for mothers of families, to be provided with a thing like this, which is at once so safe and so efficacious. If the use of this weed were generally adopted, the art and mystery of healing wounds, and of curing sprains, swellings and other external maladies, would very quickly be reduced to an unprofitable trade.

The owner of one copy of this book, R. Stibbon, has written in the front a reminder about this passage on mallows. Yet this is a remedy that, in country areas, never fell from use. I have met several people who remember its use for treating abscesses, and for bringing boils to a head.[22] One Norfolk informant related how the fruit, the 'cheeses' referred to above, were chewed by children as a laxative.[23] In Norfolk, the plant is still known as 'pick-cheese' (see p. 164). Vickery records several twentieth-century remedies using mallow, including an ointment used for sores, grazes and bruises,[24] although its use as a wound-healer is not recorded by Pechey in his *Herbal* of 1694. Mallow receives no mention at all in the British Herbal Pharmacopoeia of 1983. Other twentieth-century works on herbalism imply that its use has been superseded by marshmallow (*Althaea officinalis*) (a demulcent), and no reference had been found in the herbalist literature to its use in treating wounds. Yet mallow is a far more common plant in the wild than is marshmallow, which would explain its widespread use in traditional country remedies, and it is worth noting that its use has survived in oral tradition, but not in official herbalism.

Diaries are sometimes a source of information concerning country remedies. Richard Pococke, Bishop of Meath, undertook three tours in Scotland in the middle of the eighteenth century. In Mull he noted that, 'In this island and other parts they chew the root of an herb called charnicle, a sort of wild liquorice, and it is said when they drink whiskey it keeps them from being intoxicated.'[25] The charnicle described here is probably the same plant that is mentioned by several other eighteenth-century travellers, such as Pennant, Lightfoot and Defoe.[26] Beith identifies the plant in modern terms as *Orobus tuberosus* (now known as *Lathyvus tuberosus*), a type of vetch.[27] Bryant, in his eighteenth-century *Flora Dietetica*, describes this plant:

> The roots of this when boiled are said to be nutritious. They are held in great esteem by the Scotch Highlanders, who chew them as we do tobacco, and thus often make a meal of them; for being of a sedative nature, they pall the appetite and allay the sensation of hunger, the same as Tobacco does.[28]

Another written source of information on the practice of country medicine is provided by Floras, especially regional nineteenth-century Floras. Pigott recorded several interesting fragments of country lore in his *Flowers and Ferns of Cromer and its Neighbourhood*:

> The Yarrow Milfoil (*Achillea millefolium*) with its strong smell and white cushion of flowers tinged with pink, which has been recommended to us by the cottagers as a fine drink in cases of asthma and consumption grows here.
>
> Its neighbour, the Common Groundsel (*Senecio vulgaris*), is much used for poultices for inflamed limbs.[29]

Pennecuik, describing the flora of Tweeddale in Scotland, tells us of devil's-bit scabious (*Succisa pratensis*) that 'A strong decoction of it, continued a good while together, is an empirical secret for gonorrhoeas', knowledge which he attributes to Withering.[30]

Unfortunately, many floras, such as that by Anne Pratt,[31] give general hearsay evidence of the country uses of plants, and it is very difficult to assess the reliability of such statements, as well as impossible to relate them to specific geographical areas of usage. The acclaimed photographer Emerson not only left a remarkable visual record of the county of Suffolk, but also left notes on the country medicine practised there. His observations included blackcurrant (*Ribes nigrum*) tea for a sore throat, dandelion, pumpkin seed (*Cucurbita* sp.) or rosemary (*Rosmarinus officinalis*) tea for retention of urine; a poultice of chamomile flowers for tonsillitis or diphtheria; fresh earth mould for cuts; beating with holly (*Ilex aquifolium*) leaves for chilblains; powdered acorns (*Quercus robur*) for diarrhoea, pilewort (*Ranunculus ficaria*) for piles, crab apple (*Malus sylvestris*) juice for bruises, raw carrot or the chopped leaves of box (*Buxus sempervirens*) for worms, currant leaves applied to sore lips, parsley break stone (*Petroselinum crispum*) for gravel, a decoction of mallow leaves for strains, chickweed (*Stellaria media*) poultices for sore legs, a decoction of broom-tops (*Cytisus scoparius*) for renal diseases and dropsies 'and here the peasants are as wise as the Faculty', and pennyroyal as an emmenagogue, while the blooms of furze (*Ulex europaeus*) are made into a tea by the gipsies 'which they assert is a powerful emmenagogue'.[32]

Such examples could be multiplied, but these few will serve to illustrate the point that traditional remedies were incorporated into the literature of the day; to what extent information flowed in the opposite direction is less clear.

Obviously the wealthy would have access to all sources of information, whereas for the majority of the 'Common People', their sources of information were likely to be mainly oral. The literate and wealthy could draw on printed books, newspapers and magazines, as well as information supplied by friends or by the medical profession. For the illiterate, the only available information was that transmitted by family and friends. This explains the enormous difference between the domestic medicine of the rich and the poor, but as we have seen in the above examples, it is sometimes possible to discover examples of home remedies used by all groups of people in the manuscripts and books written by the wealthy. None of these fragments, however interesting, can supply the complete practice of domestic medicine, but they do illustrate the limited interaction between popular traditional medicine and orthodox medicine.

2. Glimpses of Traditional Plant Medicine from Ballads, Proverbs and Poetry

The fact that plant remedies formed a basic and unquestioned part of daily life has led to their incorporation in ballads, songs, proverbs and poetry, and it is worth exploring how much information, if any, can be gleaned from these sources. Of these four sources, ballads and proverbs are probably the nearest we come to written information about what was essentially an oral tradition. Ballads are themselves oral, and it is only through the diligence of recorders such as Child in Scotland that many have survived to the present day. Proverbs, too, are a part of ordinary folk culture, and as such might be expected to include the occasional snippet of information concerning traditional plant use. Folk songs, like ballads, are essentially oral and many have

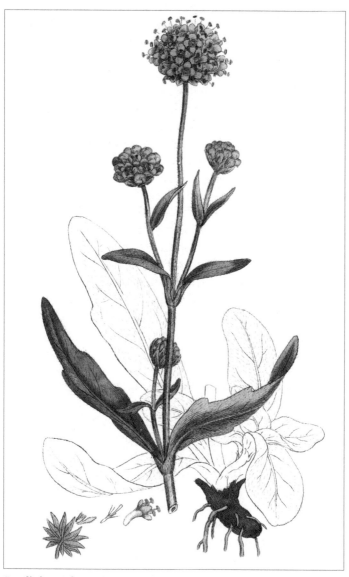

Devil's bit scabious (*Succisa pratensis*), from Sowerby's *English Botany*.
(Photograph courtesy of John Innes Foundation Historical Collections)

doubtless been lost to posterity, but again they represent the voice of the ordinary person, and include details of ordinary life. Poetry, on the other hand, was and remains the province of the privileged and literate. It deals, not with the mundane realities of sickness and disease, but with the more dramatic, emotional and aesthetic sides of man's relationship with his surroundings. One would expect it to include, not the daily uses of plants, but their more heroic aspects, and their symbolism.

The examples from English literature that follow are of interest in that they do reflect a changing attitude of people to plants; from being a source of survival, and a necessary part of daily life, they gradually become associated with magical symbolism and, in Victorian times, often became overlaid with sentimentality. There were probably very few plants in our native flora that have not been used in some way or other in the past. But because the majority of this knowledge was handed down orally, as the practices have discontinued, so has the information been lost.

Seeking for traces of this knowledge in poetry, it is logical to look back to the poetry originating in times when plant usage was at its height. Many of our ballads, though recorded in the nineteenth and twentieth centuries, have their roots further back. The early seventeenth century probably marked the heyday of the Englishman's appreciation of the countryside: at this time 'the country was the actual home of the great majority of men ... the love of nature received conscious and reiterated expression in the verses of pastoral, dramatic, epic and lyrical poets, of whom the most notable are Spenser, Shakespeare, Herrick, Marvell and Milton'.[33] The 'unlettered crowd paid the bulk of the gate money' in the audiences for plays, including Shakespeare's. References to daily life (including daily illness) had to be relevant to them.

There are innumerable references in Shakespeare's work to herbs and their uses. The sheer abundance of these references speaks for itself; herbs were a common part of common life. Naturally, many of these references are to the dramatic effects of plants:

> Not poppy, nor mandragora
> Nor all the drowsy syrups of the world,
> Shall ever medicine thee to that sweet sleep
> Which thou owed'st yesterday
>
> *Othello*, III, iii. 331

One would hardly expect the common usage of ordinary plants for common ailments to figure in heroic poetry. There is instead an emphasis on the dramatic and magical elements of plant healing, as in this charm prepared by an aged nurse in Spensers's *Faerie Queen*. She

> gathered Rew and Sauine, and the flowre
> Of Camphora, and Calamint, and Dill,
> All of which she in an earthen Pot did poure,
> And to the brim with Colt wood did it fill.[34]

Rew (*Ruta graveolens*) and sauine, or savine (*Juniperus sabina*) are, and doubtless were then, well-known abortifacients. Camphora (*Cinnamomum camphora*), has, according to one early nineteenth-century textbook of medical botany, been used to treat practically every disease.[35] Normally the oil is used; the use of the flowers is perhaps down to poetic licence. Both calamint (*Calamintha ascendens*) and coltwood (if we take this to be coltsfoot, *Tussilago farfara*) are contraindicated in a modern textbook of herbalism for use during pregnancy.

These two latter plants are the only ones mentioned in the spell that are native to Britain, and would therefore have been freely available to rich and poor alike. It is of course probable that those in both Shakespeare's and Spenser's audiences who could not afford the more exotic ingredients (such as camphor), would nevertheless have heard of them.

Another example of a reference to herbal healing is to be found in Spenser's *Faerie Queene*:

> Into the woods thenceforth in hast she went
> To seeke for hearbes, that mote him remedy;
> For she of hearbes had great intendiment,
> Taught of the Nymphe, which from her infancy
> Her nourced had in trew Nobility:
> There, whether it diuine *Tobacco* were
> Or *Panachaea*, or *Polygony*,
> She found, and brought it to her patient deare
> Who al this while lay bleeding out his hart-bloud neare
>
> The soueraigne weede betwixt two marbles plaine
> She pownded small, and did in peeces bruze,
> And then atweene her lilly handes twaine,
> Into his wound the iuyce thereof did scruze[36]

The identity of the *panachaea* must be in doubt: Smith and de Selincourt suggest that it is all heal,[37] but this name is given to a number of plants. Polygony probably refers to *Polygonum* sp. Perhaps the likeliest identity is *Polygonum bistorta*, whose roots and leaves 'had a great reputation as a remedy for wounds'.[38] Its status as a native British plant is dubious. Tobacco is certainly not a native (it was introduced to England by Sir Walter Raleigh in 1586,[39] during Spenser's lifetime). It would not have been possible to gather these plants in the woods, but poetic licence allows this! At least two out of the three ingredients would not have been generally available to the poor for first aid, so again this suggests that one can learn more about the medication of the rich than the poor from major poetic sources.

A more recent poet, Longfellow, refers to an earlier use of fennel (*Foeniculum vulgare*) in these terms:

> Above the lower plant it towers,
> The Fennel with its yellow flowers;
> And in an earlier age than ours
> Was gifted with the wondrous powers
> Lost vision to restore.

This seems to be a reference to Pliny's claim that adders used the plant to improve their eyesight; there is no reason to suppose that it formed part of British folk medicine, but the fact that it has become enshrined in poetry will probably mean that this remedy will for ever be attributed to folk medicine!

These examples might suggest that there is little information to be gleaned from the major poets concerning plant remedies used exclusively by the common people. There is, however, some information concerning contemporary medical practice, and in some instances there will of course have been overlap in the plants used by official and by traditional medicine. Any folk usage of plants that *did* find its way into famous poetry would become preserved for all time. This brings its own dangers of misinterpretation. For example, the nineteenth-century poet Clare refers to:

> Corn Poppies that in crimson dwell
> Called headaches from their sickly smell

This interpretation of the name 'headache flower' has become petrified in the literature[40] (see p. 108), yet it is probably a complete misinterpretation. At least in Norfolk, and probably elsewhere too, the plant has been used within living memory as a *cure* for headache, especially for hangovers.[41]

Poetry *is* a major source of information concerning the magical associations of plants; this is not surprising, since magic of all kinds holds a strong appeal, and is the very stuff of poetry. This has resulted in the magical usage of plants being greatly over-stressed, simply because it is over-represented in the literature. Much of what was probably written for entertainment has been taken as evidence of the credulity of man (especially of the poorer classes), and has given the whole subject of herbal medicine an overtone of witchcraft and superstition that it does not deserve. Here are some examples of ballads recorded by Child where the plants mentioned have apparently magical qualities:

> Can you make me a cambrick shirt
> Parsley, sage, rosemary and thyme
> Without any seam or needle work?
> And you shall be a true lover of mine.[42]

Nobody was meant to believe that the plants mentioned actually had these magical qualities, but they make for an entertaining story! Similarly, in 'The Ballad of King Estmere' we read (but are not expected to believe!):

> My mother was a westerne woman
> And learned in gramarye
> And when I learned at the schole
> Something shee taught itt mee

> There growes an hearbe within this field,
> And if it were but knowne,
> His color which is whyte and red,
> It will make blacke and browne
>
> His color, which is browne and blacke
> It will make redd and whyte;
> The sworde is not in all Englande
> Upon his coate will byte.[43]

But the Victorians were guilty of embroidering such associations of plants with magic, creating a pseudo-folklore connected with plants. 'The Witch's Ballad' by William Bell Scott (1812–90) illustrates the exaggerated associations of plants with magic and witchcraft:

> Our hair with marigolds was wound
> Our bodices with love-knots laced
> Our merchandise with tansy bound ...
>
> Each one in her wame shall hide
> Her hairy mouse, her wary mouse
> Fed on madwort and agramie.[44]

Agramie (agrimony, *Agrimonia eupatoria*), as well as having magical associations, has been and continues to be used in mundane country medicine, as a treatment for lumbago, a spring-time tonic, and a urinary stimulant:[45] I have also come across its use in East Anglia for jaundice, rheumatism and lumbago.[46] Such practical uses do not fire the imagination in the way that magical ones do. An old English manuscript states of agrimony:

> If it be leyd under mann's heed,
> He shall sleepyn as he were deed;

> He shall never drede ne wakyn
> Till fro under his heed it be takyn.[47]

It is my own opinion that such statements were never meant to be taken seriously; rather they were a way of enlivening a medical text.

Sometimes the poets got it right, sometimes they did not: poetry, after all, is not meant to be strictly factually accurate. Writing of cowslips (*Primula veris*), Coleridge tells us:

> What time the fairies made them orbs of green
> And gave to every herb mysterious power,
> Thou wast the chosen crest of Elfin Queen,
> Her banner tall in battle's perilous hour.

This does not strictly tell us anything more about the cowslip, but it does serve to illustrate an important point. Since the mode of action of plants in medicine was largely unknown, it *was* mysterious. Cowslips, especially in the form of cowslip wine, have been and continue to be used as a valuable sedative. In the words of Pope:

> For want of rest
> Lettuce and Cowslip wine *probatum est.*[48]

The so-called 'Language of Flowers' was another Victorian invention by the upper classes. As Vickery has pointed out, this language 'was an entirely literary tradition which had little, if any, influence on the "folk".'[49]

If we wish to glean information concerning the common remedies used by the illiterate, it is to oral traditions that we must look. One would expect to find more references to commonly used plants within such oral traditions as ballads and proverbs but the very ordinariness of well-known plant remedies probably militates against their inclusion in ballads, which were stories told for pleasure, and unlikely to emphasize the ordinary aspects of life.

However, there is an occasional reference to be found, as in the story of the Queen's Maries. Several versions of this ballad have survived. Mary Queen of Scots conferred the name Mary (or Marie) on each of her ladies-in-waiting. When Marie Hamilton discovered she was pregnant by the king, she knew that the queen would have her put to death, unless she could bring about an abortion:

> The king is to the Abbey gane
> To pu' the Abbey Tree
> To scale the babe frae Marie's heart
> But the thing it wadna be.[50]

In another version of the same ballad, recorded by Child in Motherwell, from an 1825 recitation, Marie herself gathers the plant:

> She's gane to the garden gay
> To pu of the savin tree
> But for a' that she could say or do
> The babe it would not die.[51]

The Abbey Tree is another name for savine, or juniper, of which the physician John Pechey wrote in 1694, 'It forces the courses and causes miscarriage, upon which account they are too well known and too much used by wenches.'[52] Jamieson's *Scottish Dictionary* tells us that the saving tree (or sabine) is said to kill the foetus in the womb. 'It takes its name from this, as being able to save a young woman from shame. This is what makes gardeners and others wary about giving it to females.'[53] In Somerset, in the present century, another species of juniper (*Juniperus communis*) is known by the brutally clear name of Bastard Killer.[54] Unfortunately for the Queen's Marie, the juniper failed to make her abort, and the Queen had her executed in the Tolbooth.

Savin was probably used by people of all classes as an abortifacient, and was not exclusive to traditional medicine. The conspiracy of silence that surrounds the subject of abortion even today has limited the number of abortifacients I could discover when researching plant remedies used in East Anglia within living memory. Even though abortion was probably one of the few means of contraception available in rural areas, right up to the beginning of the twentieth century, the natural reticence of people on the subject means that it is more usual to find a fleeting reference, as in the ballad of Tam Lin:[55]

> There grows an herb in Carterhaugh
> Will twine you an the bairn.

What the herb was, we are not told. So often, there is silence on this subject. An old Devon rhyme hints at possible use of another plant in contraception or abortion:

> Boy's Love is Maiden's Ruin
> But half of it is her own doing.

'Boy's Love' and 'Maiden's Ruin' are Devon names for southernwood, *Artemisia abrotanum*. In Devon in the twentieth century, the plant has been claimed to procure abortion, used as an infusion.[56]

It is an irony that, as Riddle has pointed out, one of the richest sources of information on abortifacient plants is monastic writings, where they are frequently mentioned

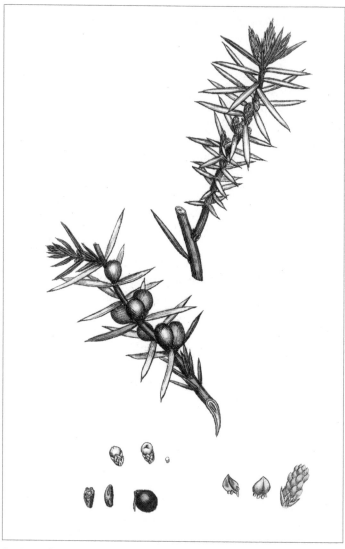

Juniper (*Juniperus communis*), from Sowerby's *English Botany*.
(Photograph courtesy of John Innes Foundation Historical Collections)

in a cautionary way, as unsuitable for use during pregnancy.[57] Similar negative information has continued to be provided in many herbal books right up to the present day. Under the heading of plants used to treat amenorrhoea there are many plants with undoubted abortifacient properties.[58]

There are thus several reasons why poetry is a poor source of information concerning common traditional plant remedies: daily illness is not a suitable subject for poetry, unless it has a heroic aspect. Poetry in general is available only to the literate class. Lastly, the writers of poetry may themselves be unaware of the daily plant remedies used by their social inferiors. For all these reasons, only small scraps of information can be obtained.

Proverbs seem to present a different picture. They are everyday sayings and, by definition, will have been used by rich and poor alike. They refer to daily events and experiences, and do not pretend to any literary merit. In effect, they are pieces of oral history, preserved in the spoken word, and sometimes in the written word. Usually they are impossible to date with any accuracy, but this does not detract from their value as sources of information for common observations or beliefs. Here are some examples of proverbs that are fragments of now largely-forgotten knowledge or beliefs concerning plants:

> March wind-flowers, so frail and pure
> Keep all infection from your door

> Beware of St Anthony's turnips
> (*i.e. roots of buttercup*)

> Vervain and dill
> Hinders witches from their will

Gather Sweet-briar in June, for it promoteth cheerfulness (*Scotland*)

He that sleepeth under a walnut tree doth get to himself pains in the head

Lightning never strikes an elder tree

Pluck the fruit of the Rowan and put witches to flight

These are all taken from a book of country lore,[59] and the main source given is a handwritten collection of lore belonging to the grandmother of a friend of the author, so it is impossible to guess at their age or origins. They are tiny fragments of once widespread country knowledge, beliefs, and humour. So much of this knowledge is disappearing fast, and is likely to die out with the present generation of elderly country people. As a part of our heritage, such information surely deserves to be recorded for posterity:

> He that would live for aye
> Must eat sage in May.

is another proverb of unknown origin.[60] A seventeenth-century proverb recorded by Aubrey tells us:

> Eat Leekes in Lide and ramsins in May
> And all the yeare after physitians may play.[61]

Ramsins, or ramsons is the country name for *Allium ursinum*, still eaten as a vegetable, and used within living memory for coughs and colds.[62] Leeks likewise have been roasted and eaten as a cough and cold cure within living memory in East Anglia.[63] A Channel Island version of this proverb runs: 'Eate leekes with sorye (sorrel) in March, cresses in April, Ramsons in May and all ye yeare after ye phisitions may goe play'.[64] This is probably even better advice, since the vitamin-C rich cress and sorrel (*Rumex acetosa*) would have been a good antidote to scurvy, after the long winter with few vegetables available.

An old saying, again of unknown origin, claims 'Drink Motherwort and live to be a continuous source of continuous astonishment and grief to waiting heirs.'[65] Gerard tells us that 'some woman poet or other' made these verses:

> They that will have their heale
> Must put Setwall in their Keale

Setwall is the country name for valerian (*Valeriana officinalis*), still widely used by herbalists today to promote sleep and allay pain.[66]

The scarlet pimpernel (*Anagallis arvensis*), until recently a common weed of our cornfields, but now largely sprayed out of existence, was much more highly prized by our ancestors. An old English proverb claims:

> No heart can think, no tongue can tell,
> The virtues of the pimpernel.[67]

Recommended by Gerard for dim sight, the plant is still used in folk medicine in this country, for treating sore eyes and for stings.[68]

A country rhyme records the use in the past for sloes (the fruit of blackthorn, *Prunus spinosa*):

> At the end of October go gather up sloes,
> Have thou in readiness plenty of those,
> And keep them in bedstraw or still on the bough
> To stay both the flux of thyself and thy cow.[69]

Today, the plant is used only for making sloe gin and walking sticks, although there are twentieth-century records of the use of sloes for treating warts, and as a gargle for sore throats and for whooping cough.[70] The following saying is of unknown origin, but claimed to be of great antiquity:

> Get water of fumiter liver to cool
> And other the like, or go die like a fool.[71]

Fumitory (*Fumaria* sp.) has been used as a cosmetic in recent times. In Wiltshire it was known as Fevertory.[72]

'Sell your coat and buy Betony' is an old proverb that needs little explanation. The physician Turner recounts thirty complaints such as that can be cured by betony (*Stachys officinalis*), and then tells us: 'I shall conclude with the words I have found in an old manuscript ... More than all this have been proved of Betony.'[73] In the twentieth century, betony tea was known to be used for headaches[74] and kidney complaints (see p. 118), but there remain few traces of its other uses in folk medicine.

3. Evidence from Plant Names

> That which we call a rose
> By any other name would smell as sweet.

If we accept that traditional plant remedies in Britain are part of a primarily oral tradition, then it follows that a full written record of them will not be available for the twentieth century, let alone for earlier times, although some glimpses can be obtained from manuscripts and printed sources. Another avenue to explore is the naming of plants used in the past for food and medicine. Starting from today's country names for native British plants, is it possible to glean information concerning their earlier usage? For instance, 'dishyluggs' or coltsfoot, mentioned in Chapter 2 (p. 64), is known in Somerset by the more transparent name of 'baccy plant'.[75]

Another example of a country name of great antiquity faithfully preserved by oral tradition concerns a plant that has never been prominent in mainstream medicine. One of its English names is goosegrass: to botanists it is *Galium aparine*. I have been told of various traditional uses for the plant: it has been fed to poultry, as the name goosegrass implies; the small prickly fruit have been roasted and used as a coffee substitute; the whole plant has been used in the spring to make a tonic drink; and the fresh plant has been used in the treatment of a variety of skin conditions. While talking to an elderly gipsy lady, I asked her whether she recalled any uses of the plant from her youth. For a long time she could not make out what plant I was referring to: when she recognized it, she referred to it as hayriff. This name is recorded in the forms 'heyreve' and 'heyrive' in a collection of Anglo-Irish receipts copied around 1300.[76] My informant had never learnt to read or write; presumably this name had been passed down orally, with quite remarkable continuity. Grieve suggests the origin of the name as '"hedge rife", meaning taxgatherer or robber 'from its habit of plucking the sheep as they pass near a hedge'.[77] The same author records no fewer than fifteen country names for this plant.

These two anecdotes illustrate both the multiplicity of plant names in use in this country and their continuity over time. They further illustrate the varying origins of these country names. Some are traceable back to early times, as hayreve above, while others, such as dishyluggs, are secondarily derived from the botanical name. An in-depth study of all these country names, although a

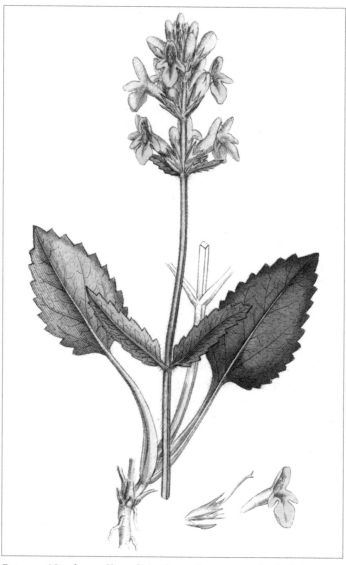

Betony (*Stachys officinalis*), from Sowerby's *English Botany*.
(Photograph courtesy of John Innes Foundation Historical Collections)

mighty task, might well bring to light otherwise forgotten uses of plants.

Whether it is possible to identify in modern botanical terms the plant or plants used in a particular remedy is a vexed question, and one that has provoked considerable argument. It does seem logical to suggest that, whatever name was given to a plant used in a traditional remedy, the *user* knew to which plant he was referring. In this respect, there was a considerable difference between the empirical user of plant remedies, and the authors of manuscripts and learned treatises and herbals. The authors may or may not have been sure of the identity of the plants of which they wrote. The users on the other hand had an extremely strong motive, namely survival, for identifying correctly the plant used in a remedy. The cultural and educational gulf between the users of country remedies and the people who wrote about these plants has probably been widened by the process of scientific taxonomy which, although obviously furthering the development of botany as a science, may also have had the side-effect of widening this gulf. This means that the modern ethnobotanist, attempting to record for posterity the uses of a particular flora, has the added challenge of learning the local country names of the plants concerned. At least twentieth-century ethnobotany has had the advantage that it is usually possible to identify the plant subject of a remedy by being shown a sample of the plant used. The historian of ethnobotany does not have this advantage. The nearest he can get to establishing the identity of a particular plant is at best an inspired guess based upon knowledge of both common and local country names of plants, together with any more strictly botanical information provided in the recipe.

In searching for possible written sources of information concerning early plant names, one could argue that manuscripts where the vernacular plant name is indicated suggest derivation of remedies from the folk tradition. Hunt has provided information on the medieval names of British plants derived from manuscript sources belonging to the twelfth and thirteenth centuries, pointing out that many names of plants attributed to the sixteenth century are actually much earlier and can be found in medieval manuscripts. Eighty-nine names attributed in the *Oxford English Dictionary* to the sixteenth century are present in medieval lists of herbs, while five hundred names found in medieval lists are not mentioned at all in the *OED*! Among the earliest recorded names for British plants, he lists many which are of Middle English and Anglo-Norman origin. Among them are names that are still clearly recognizable to the modern eye, for example 'centorie', sanicle, scammony, 'chykenmete, vyolette, wylde tesle, stychewert, plantyne, southernewode, popi'.[78]

While these are familiar to us as the country names of plants, their strict identification, particularly down to species level, is virtually impossible. For example, centorie is presumably *Centaurium* sp. Which species is referred to is impossible to determine, though one can hazard a guess that if the recipe concerned was actually used, then since the manuscript is Irish in origin, it is likely that the common centaury, *Centaurium erythraea*, would have been used since the lesser centaury (*Centaurium pulchellum*) is absent from much of Ireland. Even this cannot be established as fact, since so little is known about the earlier distribution of our native flora. Indeed, Voigts suggests that climatic differences in the past could mean that present-day Mediterranean species would have flourished in Anglo-Saxon Britain. She argues that the presence in recipes of foreign plants does not necessarily mean that such remedies were not used in practice in Anglo-Saxon Britain, and points out that two plants, woad (*Isatis tinctoria*) and Mediterranean peony (*Paeonia mascula*), were both cultivated in England during Anglo-Saxon times, and are both mentioned as remedies in Anglo-Saxon remedy books.[79]

The other early plant names mentioned above are clearly identifiable, at least as far as the genus. Sanicle is still used today for *Sanicula europaea*. Scammony, *Convolvulus scammonia*, is not a native bindweed, but can be grown here on dry soils,[80] and may or may not have been imported from Syria for its medicinal use in the thirteenth century. Chykenmete, as chicken's meat, is a name still used in East Anglia for chickweed, *Stellaria media*.[81] The name vyolette could refer to any of the native species of violet (*Viola odorata, V. riviniana, V. reichenbachiana*, etc.), several of which have been used in the past in both official and traditional medicine. Wylde tesle needs no explanation, as the teazle (*Dipsacus fullonum*). Stychewert, in the form stitchwort, today refers to *Stellaria holostea*, plantyne could be any of the genus *Plantago*, or it could refer to the unrelated *Alisma plantago-aquatica*. Southernwode probably refers to the non-native *Artemisia abrotanum*, grown as a garden plant. Popi may refer to the native *Papaver rhoeas*, or to the non-native opium poppy, *Papaver somniferum*.

This small sample of early plant names will serve to show that there is significant continuity in country names for plants, but that their identity in modern botanical terms is often impossible to establish with certainty. However, it should be emphasized again that this does not imply that the *users* of plant remedies did not know precisely which plant they intended to use.[82] Names are an important means of recognition even in illiterate societies. In the past, country people had names for each other that reflected people's role in the community; hence our present surnames Smith, Cooper, etc. In Wales and in Ireland even today, people are often known by their job as well as their name (Mick the Pub, etc.). In an age when people were much closer to and more dependent upon the countryside in which they lived, plants had a central role to play in survival: as food, medicine, bedding, roofing, to name but a few of their uses. Presumably names would have evolved which reflected a plant's usefulness to man. There would have been no 'system' to these country names, any more than there was a system to the names given to animals or indeed to objects. The names were simply a way of referring to a particular plant, and as long as a name was recognized within a community, this was all that was required of it. It is not surprising to find then that the same plant has been known by a wide variety of names at different periods of time, and in different geographical areas. Moreover, the same name may denote different plants according to the time and place of its usage. All this makes the job of identification of a particular plant used in a particular way extremely difficult. We have to appreciate that the common names of plants are just that: they represent an experience held in common by a particular community at a particular time. Such names do not have the exclusiveness of our modern scientific names. They served a completely different function. There was no classification as such: plants would have been named in response to their impact on man: the names given to plants would reflect their different uses, rather than any particular feature of the plant.

Because the earliest written accounts of plants are written by the well-educated rather than the ordinary plant user, as soon as plant names began to appear in writing they were Latinized. Not only in Britain and Europe, but presumably all over the world, man's earliest naming of plants remains unrecorded; only vestiges of early names remain. Once the written record takes over, oral names are largely lost, at least in the literature. The history of botany therefore remains almost exclusively the history of *learned* botany, leaving the common experience of hands-on use of plants side-lined and largely forgotten. Although many writers have recognized the knowledge possessed by early man, there is no direct access to this information. The best we can hope for are glimpses, such as those implied in the earliest recorded names. Even here, emphasis is largely on the early learned names:

> The herb-gatherers or rhizotomi of antiquity undoubtedly possessed a wide acquaintance with plants having reputed medicinal value. Thus when we speak in English of anemones, asparagus, crocuses, cyclamens, delphiniums, gentians, lilies, peonies, roses, violets, etc., we use names which have come to us with little or no change from the everyday speech and herbalist jargon of ancient Rome and Magna Graecia.[83]

Stearn points out that the Romans possessed many words relating to conspicuous plant structures, *notably those of economic use* (my italics), even though they failed to name the parts of the flower that were to prove later the basis of morphological taxonomy.[84] The distinction between plants used for food (and medicine) and those for timber, building, shelter was a natural one to make. This could have been the basis of the distinction between woody trees and herbs that so bedevilled early taxonomic botanists, and was not shed until the time of Linnaeus.

Indeed, in man's early development, only those plants important to him in some way would merit the recognition of a name of their own. Obvious categories of importance would be plants that provide food or shelter for people and later for their animals. Plants discovered to be harmful to people would merit recognition, too. If it were possible to trace the earliest plant names, one would probably find that they were given to plants used as food, shelter, medicine or poison. Not only would the earliest plant names have been entirely oral, they would also have been exclusive to one community.

While there is little hope of recovering the earliest names for plants, those that are first recorded in writing can in some instances shed light on their past uses. Hunt, emphasizing the fact that one name was often used for a variety of different plants with the same usefulness to people, claims that 'sanguinarie' was used to describe several plants with blood-staunching properties.[85] Like all other aspects of man's relationship with his environment, the naming of plants by early man was an entirely empirical affair. However, one can postulate that the earliest plant names are the likeliest ones to yield clues as to the uses of these plants. Where their use has been continuous, the early names have in some cases survived. One could also argue that those plants most useful to man would have received the largest number of local names, and that the multiplicity of names could also be an indicator of their usefulness.

Early monastic writings sometimes include references to local names for medicinal plants, but obviously such writings will only refer to those plants used by the monks in medicine; their pharmacopoeia will have been different to that of the country people, even though there was probably some overlap. Hunt suggests that the medieval writers had very little first-hand knowledge of the plants they were reading and writing about, when they were referring to ancient sources, and the flora of the

Mediterranean and the Near East.[86] The situation was probably better where native plants were concerned. Voigts quotes the French ninth-century monastic cultivator of plants, Walahfrid Strabo, who, though speaking of Richenau, describes a situation that probably applied in Anglo-Saxon Britain too. Speaking of his own knowledge of plants, he tells us:

> This I have learnt not only from common opinion
> And searching about in old books, but from experience –
> Experience of hard work and sacrifice of many days
> When I might have rested, but chose instead to labour.[87]

Here is first-hand evidence of the way in which common knowledge was incorporated into the learned tradition. With the passage of time, the copying and re-copying of manuscripts, and the multiplicity and inaccuracy of the names used for plants, it is not surprising to find it impossible to disentangle the truly folk plant remedies from those of officialdom.

It could be argued that early monastic writings, as opposed to those of lay scholars, are likeliest to incorporate endemic knowledge of local medicinal plants. Monasteries traditionally cared for the social outcasts as well as the chronically sick, and there was probably more communication between monks and the ordinary country people than there would have been between the lay learned and the ordinary person. Morton points out that in some instances, at least, monks were aware that the plants they used in medicine were not those of the ancients, and they sometimes included vernacular names for the local plants that they used medicinally:

> The monks learnt, and no doubt used, the virtues of local herbs – knowledge from which the wealthy town physician

was cut off – and realized that the plants they gathered and grew were different from the simples of official medicine.

It thus came about that local plants were sporadically added to the classical herbals; sometimes a familiar plant was substituted for an unknown Mediterranean herb under the old classical name, leading to increased confusion, but in other cases the vernacular name was put in to show a genuine addition.[88]

The picture was further confused, though, by the invention of new vernacular names for some plants; many of these were 'christianized' names, such as herba St Joannis for *Hypericum perforatum*.[89] In the tri-lingual manuscripts of thirteenth-century England, some plants are referred to by Latin, English and Anglo-Norman names. At this period, Hunt points out that 'some plants were certainly more familiar in their indigenous name forms, whilst others seem to be referred to only by their Latin names. Much of course depended on the culture of the compiler and user and the auxiliary materials at their disposal.'[90]

With the advent of the first printed herbals, native knowledge of plant usage probably became further obscured, as the authors attempted to equate the plants used in contemporary medicine with those of the ancient authorities. Many authors have pointed out the botanical inaccuracy of the largely stylized illustrations of plants in the early herbals. To what extent this actually mattered is debatable, as the writers of these herbals for the most part served a portion of the population who would depend on others to gather the plants for them. Furthermore, one could argue that many of the plants were sufficiently well-known to their users to need no illustration[91] (although in the sixteenth century Turner laments the lack of botanical knowledge among his learned contemporaries in Cambridge).[92] The first herbals to be accurately illustrated by drawings of plants from life (e.g. Fuch's herbal) began to set the botanical record straight, but by this time much native knowledge would already have been lost. Once the tradition of printed herbals was established, no other herbal authority was officially recognized, and the practice of country medicine, despite continuing up to the present day, remained undocumented.

The sixteenth-century botanist Turner recorded a number of vernacular names for the British plants he described, as well as providing anglicized names for other species, which subsequently became the common names by which these plants were known in print: some of these names, such as butcher's broom (*Ruscus aculeatus*), have become accepted as the country names by which these plants are known in print; whether such 'secondary' country names were ever adopted by those who actually used the plants in rural medicine is extremely difficult to establish. In many ways it is surprising that some of the vernacular names given by Turner are still in use as country names today: names such as kingcuppe (*Caltha palustris*), water plantane (*Alisma plantago-aquatica*), rocket, butterbur (*Petasites hybridus*), butcher's broom, mullen (*Verbascum thaspus*), sauce alone (*Alliaria peiolata*), daffodil (*Narcissus pseudo-narcissus*), horsetail (*Equisetum* sp.), alexanders (*Smyrnium olusatrum*), horehound (*Marrubium vulgare*), yarrow (*Achillea millefolium*) and whin are all still used as they were when Turner was the first to record them in print.[93]

As printed works proliferated, and copied from each other, it became increasingly difficult to disentangle from the names given to British plants those which were original local country names. Despite these difficulties, some at least of the earliest names have survived, and a study of these could throw some light on forgotten uses of these plants. Mullein, for example, was used in the past for treating leprosy or melanders, and this may well be the derivation of its name. It was called 'molegn' by the Anglo-Saxons, and 'malen' in Old French.[94] Continuity of naming of a plant is one parameter that could indicate its long history of usefulness, along with the possibility that the number of names could reflect its importance.[95]

With the advent of our modern system of plant classification in the sixteenth and subsequent centuries, scientific classification has largely replaced the casual empirical naming of plants useful to man. The concept of natural affinities between plants was glimpsed in the sixteenth century by botanists such as Caesalpino[96] and de l'Obel, and recognized more clearly by Kaspar Bauhin in the early seventeenth century. A classification based on plant characteristics began to replace the simple listings of plants that we find in the earlier herbals. No longer were plants described entirely for their medicinal virtues; instead, a scientific system of classification emerged, culminating in the work of Linnaeus in the eighteenth century. From his time onwards, plants were to bear the official binomial names invented by him and his successors. The new classification was based primarily on the perceived afffinities between plants. The first or generic name (*Bellis* in *Bellis perennis*) indicates the group to which the plant belongs; the second, specific, name (*perennis* in *Bellis perennis*) indicates the species to which the plant belongs; individuals of one species resemble one another and can interbreed. In this way, the common names for plants have undergone extensive revision by the learned. The binomial system of classification introduced by Linnaeus brought order to the science of taxonomy, but it has served to obscure, and in some instances abolish altogether, the earlier country names for plants.

However, the Linnaean names were in some instances based upon the properties of the plants. The daisy is a case in point. Linaeus' name of *Bellis perennis* refers to its use in Classical times as a wound healer (Latin: *bellum*, war). In instances such as these the scientific name preserves some knowledge of the plant's former use. Indeed, the specific epithet *officinalis* indicates that the plant was recognized as used in official medicine. In some cases it is possible to trace the generic name of a plant to its actual medicinal use. An example is the self-heal, whose botanical name *Prunella* is claimed to have been derived from the German 'die Breuen', an inflammation of the mouth for which it was used.[97] But such names do not necessarily reflect *folk* usage, certainly not British folk usage, and many of what today pass as country names are in fact translations of botanical names.

There are numerous examples where the Linnaean name does not in any way reflect the plant's usage; indeed, why should it? Linnaeus was concerned not with the uses of the plants but with their phylogenetic relationships. He used Latin as the accepted language of the learned, and decreed that 'Generic names which have not a root derived from Greek or Latin are to be rejected.'[98] The generic names of plants are always Latinized, but in our present era, 'may be taken from any source whatever and may even be composed arbitrarily'.[99] The scientific classification was bound to be totally unrelated to the purely empirical naming of plants by country people. The evolution of botany as a science has inevitably resulted in some information concerning plant uses being lost, along with the country names of plants.

Linnaeus was not the first person to obscure the country names of plants. Many names were Christianized by the monastic tradition: St John's wort (*Hypericum* sp.), St James wort (*Senecio jacobaea*, better known as ragwort), marigold, marygold (*Calendula officinalis*). Some country names have proved robust enough to survive the onslaught of both religion and science. Daisy (*Bellis perennis*) could be one such example, apparently derived from the Anglo-Saxon for the day's eye (dages ege), i.e. the sun, from its sun-like appearance. A few names have survived with quite remarkable continuity. The old country name for plantain (*Plantago* sp.), waybread, is clearly traceable back to Anglo-Saxon times. This plant has been used as far back as it can be traced for food and for medicine. It is tempting to speculate that those plants that were particularly useful to man would have long-lasting country names; however, against this argument, the fact that a plant was known to be useful could lead to its incorporation into the learned tradition, whether monastic or medical. In turn, this could obscure or even bury altogether the traces of earlier country names for the plant.

Examples of present-day country names that clearly indicate the use of the plant are numerous. Spindle, for example (*Euonymus europaeus*), as its name suggests, supplied the wood for making spindles. Interestingly, a west-country name for the same plant is louseberry, and at least in that part of the country, the berries have been used within living memory to treat head lice in children. This example leads on to another important point: because country names vary for a particular plant, it is possible that this variation may reflect varying usage. In Norfolk, the common field poppy (*Papaver rhoeas*) goes by the name of headache flower. As noted on p. 85, its seeds are helpful for treating headaches, especially hangovers.[100] Bird's eye (*Veronica* sp.) has the local Norfolk name of sore-eyes. The petals were infused for treating sore eyes. Probably in the distant past, names conferred upon plants were chosen to indicate their importance to man. The sixteenth-century names 'openars tre' (*Mespilus germanica*) and arsmart (*Polygonum hydropiper*) do not leave much to the imagination. From the same century, the name 'dyshwasshynges' for the horsetail (*Equisetum* sp.) clearly celebrates its usefulness as a pot scourer.

Probably food and medicine were not as separate as they are today, and many plants were used as both. Country names such as chickweed, sowbread (*Cyclamen hederifolia*), cow-wheat (*Melampyrum* spp.), fat hen (*Chenopodium album*), goosegrass all clearly indicate the use for which these plants were valued. All these plants have been used in the way their names suggest within living memory. Extrapolating backwards in time, historical studies of plant names could throw light on their earlier medical usage. Dafydd Evans has pointed out that in tracing the medical use of a plant 'it is prudent to examine first its efficacy as a "simple", i.e. the single remedy for an ailment ... for it is here that its basic medical function and possibly the explanation of its name is likeliest to be discovered'.[101] It might be equally valid to invert the process, and use the plant names themselves as an indication of early medicinal usage. Examples like these suggest that if one could trace the earliest country names for plants, one might uncover forgotten uses of them. In a sense, these early names embody the oral tradition of plant usage that has become obscured and largely replaced by the written tradition.

Country names change not only from place to place, but from one century to the next, and this adds further complications. Even in the twentieth century, the same name has been used in different areas to denote botanically unrelated species. Heal-all in Cornwall and Oxfordshire refers to the plant *Valeriana officinalis*, while in Northern Ireland it refers to the unrelated *Sedum telephium*. The name 'snake flower' refers to no fewer than eight different species, while 'sweethearts' refers similarly to eight unrelated species.[102] Undoubtedly, this pluralism of names was also a problem in the past, though any name serving one community and recognized within it would be adequate for the needs of that community. As Stannard points out 'the failure to appreciate ... the Latinized Greek names of many herbs did not prevent the practice of herbalism at the domestic level'.[103] If we are to recover some of the lost threads of this domestic medicine through a study of early plant names, much more research will be needed.[104]

4. Oral Testimony

When George Ewart Evans began to record the memories of villagers where he lived in Suffolk, oral history as a discipline was in its infancy. Since then, it has become widely recognized as a valuable resource in studying the recent past. This is not the place to undertake a detailed assessment of the techniques of oral history, but before considering it as a source of information on folk medicine, it is necessary to establish its general reliability.

In my own experience, oral evidence seems to be remarkably accurate when it deals with first-hand recollections. On p. 23 the example of the use of comfrey root by Romanies is mentioned. There is often a difficulty in communication, especially where plant names are concerned. This is not because the user is unclear over what plant he or she is describing: instead, it reflects the gulf between the user of the country remedy and the recorder. The latter, like myself, is likely to be a botanist, concerned with accurate botanical identification of the plant. The former will be using a country name for the plant. An example of the kind of difficulty this poses is the story of a Welshman who wrote to me concerning a plant much used in Wales for treating, among other things, earache. He gave the Welsh name of the plant, which meant nothing to me. He described the plant, but I was still unable to identify it. I sent through the post botanical illustrations of plants that I thought matched up with his description. None of them was the plant in question. Finally, in desperation, he sent me a sample of the plant, roots, earth and all. It turned out to be the houseleek (*Sempervivum tectorum*), a plant very widely used in country medicine.

This was an ideal situation; the identity of the plant was no longer in doubt. Obviously, it is desirable to always have this degree of certainty concerning the identity of a plant used in a country remedy. Unfortunately, even when remedies are recorded that have been used within living memory, such certainty is not always possible. One informant wrote to me concerning a small bush that grew in her garden when she was a child. She called it a 'sovereigne' tree. Another example of the difficulty of identification is the 'campher' root used by the relative of a Yorkshire lady to heal a deep cut when she was small (see p. 151). The informant is certain that the plant was not comfrey, but cannot provide another identity. On p. 187 the story of an ointment made from marsh dock roots is described; the land where this took place has now been drained, so one cannot ascertain whether the plant used was the 'true' (in botanical terms) marsh dock (*Rumex palustris*) or not.

These are the exceptions. In general, it *is* possible to identify with reasonable certainty the plant used in a country remedy within living memory. In fact the level of consistency among oral remedies is impressive. I am not referring here to records in the literature. Recorders of folklore, more commonly even than in other areas of research, tend to copy each other's (often unsubstantiated) records: on further scrutiny half a dozen records in the literature may sometimes be traced to a single source. But where orally recorded remedies are concerned, there is often total agreement between different informants and, in the case of the commonest plant remedies, it is easy to become tired of hearing them again and again. However, such repetition should not be ignored, since it presumably reflects the commonness of the original remedy, and the frequency with which it was used in the past. Since remedies that fall into disuse are less likely to be remembered, frequency of a particular remedy among oral records could also indicate that it has been used in the recent past.

In attempting to give the reader a taste of the kind of traditional plant remedies recorded orally in East Anglia, it is difficult to know where to start. It certainly came as a surprise to me to discover just how rich a source of information oral history could be, even in the late twentieth century, an era with few practitioners of traditional medicine. After I had worked in Norfolk for several years, I was one day walking the dog along a country footpath. I was struck by the fact that, as I looked around me, practically every plant I could see had been used in remedies in the recent past. The couch grass (*Agropyron repens*), that plague of gardeners, has been used, and indeed is still currently used, as an infusion to treat chronic cystitis.[105] The leaves of the plantain on which I was treading (*Plantago major*) were used to treat insect bites and stings.[106] The ivy leaves in the hedgerow were used to treat burns,[107] as well as corns; they were also fed to livestock when they were off-colour.[108] Blackberry leaves (*Rubus fruticosus*) were chewed for headache,[109] as well as being fed to rabbits for 'pod belly'.[110] The milky juice from dandelions was rubbed on to warts, [111] and even the holly leaves were used by the stoical East Anglians to beat chilblains until they bled (presumably a drastic-sounding way of improving the circulation).[112] Stinging nettles (*Urtica dioica*), growing in profusion beside the path, were used in innumerable ways: made into soup and puddings,[113] or springtime beer;[114] given to treat anaemia;[115] fed to livestock;[116] and used both internally as an infusion and externally as a counter-irritant to allay the pain of rheumatism.[117] The juice was even squeezed into the ear for earache; while in Suffolk it was used to treat the sting inflicted by the leaves![118] Even the bryony (*Bryonia dioica*), twining up the hawthorn (*Crataegus monogyna*) hedge, figured in a plant remedy. My informant told me that it was known to be poisonous, but the berry was used to squeeze on to chilblains.[119] The sweet-smelling honeysuckle flowers (*Lonicera* spp.) were made into an infusion to treat asthma,[120] and the fallen acorns under my feet had in the past been ground up and boiled in milk to treat diarrhoea.[121] There were patches of chickweed (*Stellaria media*) growing beside the path, which I had recently been told could be made into a poultice to treat skin rashes.[122] It occurred to me that one of the very few common plants around me that seemed not to have been used in country remedies was the abundant cow parsley (*Anthriscus sylvestris*). A few days later I was told by an elderly lady how she used to treat laminitis in horses with a hot infusion of cow parsley![123] These are only a small fraction of the collection of plant remedies with which oral history had provided me, in a short space of time and a selected area. They serve to illustrate what a rich and important source this is.

Another feature of oral history that I had not appreciated until I began this work is the speed with which it takes one back into the past. Virtually all of my informants were elderly. In some instances they had been brought up by grandparents. In these cases, the childhood remedies they described belonged to the early nineteenth century. An even more dramatic example came from a man, now in his sixties and living in Norfolk, but brought up by his grandmother in Scotland. He recalled tales his granny had told him about her own grandmother (see p. 166). In this very real way, oral history brings the past to life.

There is obviously more validity in recording plant remedies directly from the users of them, rather than seeking information in the literature. Unfortunately, in present-day Britain the users of traditional country remedies are very few and far between. The knowledge of such remedies rests in the minds of people now in their eighties and nineties, and in very few instances have they passed on their knowledge to the next generation. Perhaps they do not see it as important; perhaps they are afraid of being seen as old-fashioned. There is an urgent need to record this information for posterity, before it is too late. Currently, members of the Institute of Medical Herbalists are setting up a network of recorders all over the country, in an effort to document traditional plant remedies throughout Britain. Surely such work deserves recognition and support, but so far it has proved very difficult to obtain either. Funding is forthcoming for ethnobotanical studies in the tropical rainforest, but we have not yet studied our own backyard plants in this way! No thorough ethnobotanical work has yet been done on native British plants; the little information we have is fragmentary, and often anecdotal. To be of maximum value to future generations, such material needs to be compiled in a thorough and systematic way, and ideally to be accompanied by voucher specimens of the plant under consideration.[124]

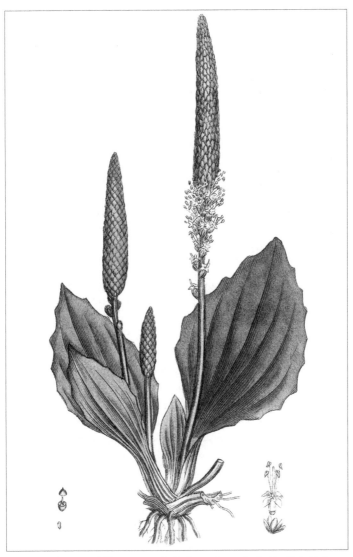

Greater plantain (*Plantago major*), from Sowerby's *English Botany*. (Photograph courtesy of John Innes Foundation Historical Collections)

As far as the accuracy of oral history as a research tool is concerned, this depends in part on whether the informant is a first-hand user of the remedy, or whether the information is hearsay, or indeed heard (or misheard!) from others, or from books. Where remedies are first-hand, they are generally accurate. Ewart Evans, when he settled in a small Suffolk village, discovered what a fund of information resided in the memories of the villagers. He became a pioneer of oral history in this country. In his writing, he stressed the accuracy of people's memories where their life work is concerned.[125] Plant remedies in the past could make a significant difference to people's lives and comfort; occasionally they could even be life-saving, though this was probably more true in past centuries than in our own. Knowledge that is important will be remembered accurately. Knowledge that has fallen from use will become increasingly cloudy. For these reasons it is important to record, not only the remedy, but if possible its context, and whether the informant has had first-hand experience of its use.

Recollections of elderly people on the subject of plant remedies often consist of a mixture of remedies that they actually used in their youth, and others that were told to them, or which they have subsequently read about. It is not always possible to separate these categories. Here is an example of an ideal letter from the oral historian's point of view. A sample of the plant was enclosed. 'My grandfather told me the "milk" from this weed would cure warts and I have found he was right.' The weed referred to was a spurge, *Euphorbia peplus*.[126] In the following example, too, there is all the data required:

> I had seven children and I had four of them down together with it (whooping cough) and I got a Swede turnip and sliced it and on every layer I put Demerara sugar and put

them on a deep soup plate and lit the oven and simmered it for a couple of hours and then gave them the liquid to drink, that soon got them well again.

This letter was from a lady in West Derby, but the same remedy has been recorded frequently in East Anglia.[127] The following example too is obviously authentic, and gives details of the plant, as well as how it was used:

I would like to tell you what my mother used to do before the War. The White Madona Lily (*Lilium candidum*) she used to gather the white petals put them in a jar then cover them with Brandy, when we used to cut ourselves she put one of the petals on the cut and cover with a Bandage it used to tingle a bit But it healed it up.[128]

Subsequently I received numerous records of this remedy, mostly from Suffolk, and a few from Norfolk. Many of them were not recalled as clearly as this; the type of lily used, the part of the plant, etc. were forgotten. Sadly, this is often the case with the oral history of plant remedies. Present knowledge is incomplete and, unless it is preserved, all knowledge will soon be lost. The following letters illustrate this point vividly:

I know of a plant which grew on a neighbour's roof and which my mother used to put on cuts – she used the leaf, which was very thick, more like a cacti – I couldn't remember name of plant, so asked an old friend and she knew at once – Houseleak (she has got a plant) but she could not tell me how it was made, she thought, a paste – and I'm afraid thats how most of them are – people can remember their parents using them, but not how the remedy was made. Everybody said the same – people all used that type of remedy, because they were quite unable to afford the Doctor – there was no health service and wages were very low.[129]

The remedies recalled by this lady include 'featherfew' for coughs, cabbage (*Brassica aleracea*) leaves put in shoes for smelly feet, rhubarb (*Rheum* x *hybridum*) leaves held on a feverish brow, chickweed boiled for boils, onions (*Allium cepa*) rubbed on stings and boiled for colds, elderberry syrup for coughs.

The writer of this next letter tells a similar story:

I am an Essex man and when I was a lad I knew quite a few of the plants that were used for different ailments but I'm afraid that I have forgotten most of them.

In the 1920s I used to collect 'Betony' for my grandfather who use to boil it and drink the water. I think this was for his kidneys or urine ... As a boy I used to chew sorrel leaves and sweet briar (*Rosa eglanteria*) and eat hips and hawes Also the new shoots of Whitethorn (*Crataegus mongyna*) which we called bread and cheese.

Ash (*Fraxinus excelsior*) leaves were also used (after boiling) for adder bites to a dog.[130]

Here is another tantalizing glimpse of incompletely remembered knowledge: 'We always had a bush named "soveriegne wood" growing in the garden which we children had to drink when the greenery was scolded, but I cannot remember the reason why.'[131]

Understandably, several informants have vivid recollections of a particular incident from their childhood:

As a small boy, I had a nasty place on my knee, which my mother was anxious about, as it would not heal. So she, I remember, took me to see my great grandmother who gave her some ointment which she had made, this I believe was home made lard, which many used in those days, this she had evidently made by using what I have always believed to be elder, boiled up, and the juice put in with the lard for it was a pale green colour. It soon cleared and healed my knee.[132]

Other examples of clearly remembered dramatic instances from the past are mentioned in Chapter 4 (e.g. severe cut, p. 151, infected foot, p. 157).

One of the most vivid stories I have been told concerns a lady now in her nineties, who has spent all her life in a small village south of Norwich. As a small child she suffered from asthma, and one day when she was four or five years old, she had a particularly severe attack. Her mother was so worried that she sent for the doctor (something that rarely happened on account of the expense). When the doctor came he held out little hope for her, but told her mother he would call again in the morning. That evening a gypsy, who was a friend of the family, called at the house and found Dolly's mother in tears. When the situation was explained, the gypsy asked for some small potatoes, which she scrubbed and boiled with their skins on. She then mashed them, skins and all, and plastered them on to pieces of sheet, with which she poultice Dolly's chest 'and I can still remember, it was as if a great weight had been lifted off my chest'. The doctor was very surprised when he called the next morning to find Dolly sitting up in bed and well again.[133]

The accuracy of such vivid memories need not be doubted, but of course many oral history records are not as complete as this. First-hand recollections are undoubtedly the best, but information gathered by other means can also provide valuable information. I have used questionnaires in schools, talks to local societies, appeals for information in the local press and on radio and television. All these methods (especially the talks on local radio) have provided very valuable information. In cases where it has been possible to follow up information provided by one individual, this has sometimes led to further information. While it is obviously ideal to record interviews on tape, this is not always possible or appropriate; in such cases, a pen and notebook must substitute. The oral history methods that I used in East Anglia are discussed more fully in my book *Country Remedies*.[134]

Despite its limitations, there can be no doubt that oral history provides invaluable information about country remedies, as well as many other topics. Indeed, as I am sure many others have found too, all kinds of unrelated but fascinating information often comes to light. I have been regaled with tales of poaching, of wherry-building in the era before mechanized boat-building, of stories of life 'below stairs'.

Ewart Evans in his own felicitous style describes this:

old men who are full of memories may be like books, but you can't open them where you like. It was best – I found – to listen and let them talk, roughly in the area where I wanted their talk to be, and then to keep them to a thread as soon as the topic I was interested in came up.[135]

Used in this way, oral history can be a delight for both the listener and the informant, as well as being a rich source of information.

3

SIMPLE PLANT REMEDIES

Characteristics of Domestic Plant Medicine

Enough examples have been given in earlier chapters of the home remedies used in Britain during the last three centuries to illustrate the type of plant remedy that has been used. At this stage it will be useful to summarize some of the characteristics of these remedies, in order that they can be compared and contrasted with both orthodox remedies and with those used by unofficial healers.

The domestic plant remedies in general used one or a few species of plants. These plants were usually either endemic or readily available as food plants (e.g. onions, cabbage, turnip (*Brassica rapa*). Rarely were the plants 'purpose-grown' as medicine. The ingredients were therefore either free or very cheap.

Contrast these features with the orthodox prescriptions in use in the eighteenth century, when polypharmacy ran wild, and Venice Turpentine, itself composed of over forty ingredients, was only one of up to thirty items in a single prescription. This difference should come as no surprise. Everybody wants value for money, and an orthodox prescription that contained only the familiar plants used in home remedies would clearly not be seen as worth paying for! Another outstanding difference between the orthodox prescriptions and the home remedies is that the former usually included foreign plant species, as well as exotic animal ingredients. In *The Druggist's Shop Opened*, printed in 1693, there are approximately 300 pages of plant remedies. There are also more than 600 pages of animal and mineral remedies, many of them weird and wonderful.[1] Although this may be an extreme example, it does serve to underline the real difference that existed between home remedies and official medicine. None of this is surprising, when home remedies are regarded as simple first-aid measures, but it is worth emphasizing simply because such a false picture is often painted of so-called folk medicine. It seems essential to separate out, from the jumble of fact and fiction that passes as folk medicine in the literature, the actual remedies that were in daily use in this country. When this is done, what emerges is not a mix of superstition, myth and magic, but a common-sense list of 'simples' used as first aid.

It is part of human nature to surround anything that we do not understand, or that we fear, with an aura of mystery. As long as plants and their uses in food and medicine were a part of everyday life, their use was governed by simple rules handed down from one generation to the next. However, as soon as such common knowledge fell out of everyday use, superstition and mystery crept in. Plant remedies as they were originally used in self-medication were probably devoid of superstition, despite what many writers have claimed.[2] This is an idea that will be illustrated in the course of this chapter.

Superstitions in daily life often represent partial or incomplete knowledge of an earlier practice. Footballers who cross themselves before a football match may or may

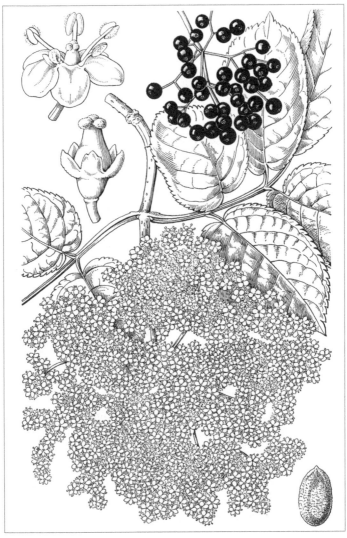

Elder (*Sambucus nigra*), from Stella Ross-Craig, *Drawings of British Plants*. (By kind permission of the Royal Botanical Gardens, Kew/ photograph courtesy of John Innes Foundation Historical Collections)

not be religious; at least in some it represents a vestige of a common daily practice of prayer. Saying 'bless you' to people when they sneeze is another example of the vestige of a religious practice, as is the practice of touching wood for good luck; this is no longer a conscious reminder of the crucifixion, but again represents the remains of an earlier widespread belief. In an analogous way, it can be suggested that many of the superstitions surrounding plants are in fact vestiges of an earlier practical use, which has now been almost forgotten. For example, it is considered unlucky by many to cut the boughs of elder, especially if they are still green (i.e. growing).[3] In past times, almost every part of the elder tree was used in some way; the taboo on cutting it could simply result from the value of this plant. Even in the relatively recent past, the list of medicinal uses for elder is impressive. The bark has been used for rheumatism,[4] the leaves for treating eczema,[5] and for making an ointment to treat burns;[6] the flowers are used as the basis of a skin lotion,[7] as well as for making wine, and the berries yield a wine with a high reputation for treating flu and colds.[8] Nowadays, such knowledge is confined to a small percentage of the population, but in the past every country dweller would have known of the uses of elder, and it was in society's interest to discourage its destruction.

Pitying reference is sometimes made to the ritual and superstition surrounding plant remedies, such as gathering the herbs in May, while the dew is on the ground, or gathering those plants that grow in shady places. Such instructions are often taken as evidence of the ignorance of the people who practised traditional medicine. In fact, this could not be further from the case. Many of these practical instructions were empirical discoveries, based on long usage of the remedies concerned. Twentieth-century science vindicates many of them. The medically active ingredients of plants are often alkaloids that vary in concentration not only with the season and time of day, but also with the habitat in which individual plants are growing.[9] Many active plant constituents peak in the morning, and in the spring, and at least in some instances it has been shown that their concentration is higher in plants grown in the shade.[10] Far from being evidence of ignorance, such instructions serve to illustrate the remarkable accuracy of some of the purely empirical findings of our forebears.

Take for example the poem often quoted by folklorists of the mermaid of the Clyde. Seeing the funeral of a young girl, she remarks:

> If they wad drink nettles in March
> And eat muggins in May
> Sae many braw maidens
> Wadna gang to clay.

Black, author of *Folk-Medicine*, written in 1883,[11] cites this as one of numerous examples of the superstitious remedies used in folk medicine. However, if we take a more careful look at it, it actually contains some excellent advice. Nettles *are* at their safest and best in March (they are actually toxic later in the year)[12]; moreover they are an excellent source of readily available iron, as well as being haemostatic (checking blood flow); they are very effective in treating anaemia resulting from heavy periods, as well as in reducing the blood loss.[13] This was probably common knowledge. The use of nettles as a springtime tonic, for both humans and animals, was widespread in Britain right up to the twentieth century (see p. 48), and traditionally the advice always included the use of the young tops of nettles.

In the diary of an eighteenth-century Surgeon apothecary living in Dalkeith, Scotland, is the following entry concerning the treatment of Mrs Turner in February 1735. She was suffering from 'fluxus mensium immodicus': 'advised to use the express'd juice of nettles which were just now in season (her courses had return'd thrice upon her since the beginning of January) also the rind of seven bitter oranges'.[14] Eighteenth- and nineteenth-century kitchen books often included nettle broth or soup.

Marian McNeill[15] gives this traditional Highland recipe:

Gather young nettles from the higher part of the wall where they are clean. Wash the tops in salted water and chop very finely. Have some good stock boiling – chicken stock is best – in which you have cooked a sufficient quantity of barley. Add the nettles, simmer till tender and season to taste.

The very frequency with which we find nettles mentioned in manuscripts and books suggests that their use was probably widespread, since like so many other home remedies, this one was probably largely handed down by word of mouth, and is therefore under-represented in the literature.

The 'muggins' mentioned by the mermaid was another plant well known for its use in treating 'women's afflictions'. Known also as mugwort (*Artemisia vulgaris* L.), this plant appears in proverbs in Scotland and Wales. Carmichael quotes:

> Wad ye let the bonny may die in your hand
> And the mugwort flowering i' the land?[16]

When I began studying plant medicines in use within living memory in Britain, mugwort did not appear at first. Then a letter from a man brought up in Essex gave this information, recalled from the 1920s: 'In our garden my father grew a clump of "Mugwort" and I think my mother used this for irregularities peculiar to women.'[17] He added that he particularly remembered the mugwort because of his father's strict instructions not to pull it up! Mugwort grows in the wild, but presumably in this case the family wished to be assured of a constant supply when it was needed.

Originally, practical instructions were part of the common knowledge of plant remedies, and would have been passed down orally from one generation of plant users to the next. Once copied into the literature of the day, they became altered in various ways. Scorn was poured on them in certain quarters, and is still today.[18] In other instances, they were altered and exaggerated, and tied in with astrology and all kinds of other beliefs. Culpeper, for example, embroidered this aspect of plant medicine.[19] There is no telling how much notice his readers took of the astrological aspect of his work, but in any case his readers represented the literate minority, and the illiterate majority doubtless continued to use plant remedies in the same way that their families had for generations. This is a further example of how the written version of plant medicine diverged increasingly from empirical traditional plant usage.

As Thompson,[20] Ewart Evans[21] and many others have testified, oral testimony is often remarkably accurate. However, once information is committed to print, any errors that creep in tend to become perpetuated, and a remarkable example of this has already been mentioned in Chapter 1 (p. 30), where the oral version of a remedy used for horses had survived accurately, whereas the printed version in a veterinary book was totally wrong. This is the kind of incorrect evidence that has often, quite unjustly, brought traditional remedies into disrepute.

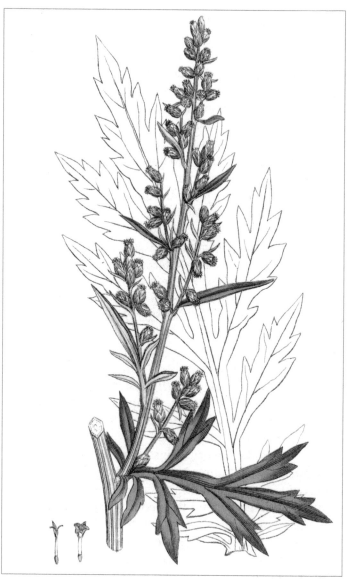

Mugwort (*Artemisia vulgaris*), from Sowerby's *English Botany*.
(Photograph courtesy of John Innes Foundation Historical Collections)

Even where the written accounts of plant remedies are not actually wrong, they are often incomplete, which can have almost as falsifying an effect. Vital instructions concerning which parts of the plant are used, or how they should be prepared, are sometimes omitted. A good example of this, mentioned in Chapter 1, is the use of comfrey, a plant used from the time of Pliny for healing sprains and fractures. Recently, its use in Britain among the middle classes has enjoyed a revival, and comfrey tea has been hailed as something of a panacea. Meanwhile, scientific studies have shown that the plant contains alkaloids that can damage the human liver, and, at least in mice, can lead to cancer.[22] This led to headlines in the press, reporting the 'Dangers of Herbal Medicines' in bold headlines. The implication was that here was a prime example of the ignorance of the people who rely on plant medicine. Yet when I was discussing plant remedies with a Romany (who, incidentally, had only learnt to read in adulthood), he was incredulous that anyone should be foolish enough to use the fresh leaves of the comfrey plant. 'Everyone knew' that you used the root of this plant as an ointment, and not the leaves as a tea.[23] The hepato-toxic alkaloids described by modern science are present in much higher concentrations in the leaves than in the root. They are poorly absorbed through the skin,[24] so used as an external application, comfrey is probably a safe remedy. No liver damage was found in twenty-nine chronic users of comfrey.[25] It seems likely that, used in the traditional way, comfrey is a valuable and relatively safe aid to healing. It should not, however, be hailed as some sort of panacea, nor should tea made from the fresh leaves be drunk in large quantities. In the field of plant remedies, as elsewhere, a little knowledge can certainly be a dangerous thing!

If it is true that plant remedies for self-use in rural England were largely devoid of myth and magic, what of those remedies that are clearly absurd? What about the acorn,[26] potato (*Solanum tuberosum*)[27] or nutmeg (*Myristica fragrans*)[28] carried in the pocket to ward off rheumatism, or the necklace of conkers (*Aesculus hippocastanum*) worn for the same purpose?[29] What of the rosehip (*Rosa canina*) carried to prevent the pain of piles?[30] Surely these would appear to be nothing other than ignorant superstitions? They are open to another interpretation. As suggested in Chapter 1 (p. 38) they could represent vestiges of earlier perfectly sensible plant remedies, now almost entirely forgotten.

If this is indeed the case, then it ought to be possible to trace the origins of these superstitions and, in some instances, this is certainly possible. Take the example of carrying a potato for rheumatism. In eighteenth-century Scotland, the water in which potatoes had been boiled was recommended, as hot as could be borne, to relieve the pain of rheumatism in the feet.[31] Grieve refers to the carrying of a potato to ward off rheumatism, but also records that 'successful experiments in the treatment of rheumatism and gout have in the last few years been made with raw potato juice ... Hot potato water has in years past been a popular remedy for some forms of rheumatism.'[32] Similarly, with the example of the necklace of conkers, an equivalent more practical version of the remedy can be found. A decoction of horse-chestnut was recorded in Essex as a traditional cure for lumbago[33] and Grieve, in her *Modern Herbal*, records the use of horse-chestnuts for treating neuralgia and sciatica.[34] It is possible that if all the records were searched exhaustively, the origins of many such plant 'superstitions' could be found in practical down-to-earth remedies. One can speculate that those plant remedies that fell earliest into disuse, and have survived only as superstitions, were the least effective in practice.

On the whole, it seems that most simple plant remedies used in self-medication throughout the centuries were largely devoid of superstition, as long as they were in current use. They were entirely practical, down-to-earth first-aid measures. If a person cut him- or herself, the immediate reaction would be to reach for a known and tried method of stopping the bleeding. Two such methods, which survived into the twentieth century, were to wrap the wound in cobwebs[35] or to make a poultice of puffballs[36, 37] or, for a smaller cut, to puff on the spores from puffballs (*Lycoperdon* sp.).[38] Although these are just the kinds of remedy that it is easy to pour scorn on and relegate to the bin of useless old wives' tales and superstitions, both have been found to be effective right up to recent times. One retired postman who had earlier in his life worked as a farm labourer recalled a friend cutting his arm seriously on a bill-hook. He shouted for cobwebs from the barn, and with these he wrapped the wound. It healed cleanly and quickly.[39] A dramatic incident was recalled by a lady living in Hemsby. As a child, she was walking her dog in some woodland when it gashed its leg badly. She picked it up, wrapped the leg as best she could and hurried to her uncle's house. By this time the dog was weak from blood loss. Her uncle fetched a bulfer (puffball) from the woods, chopped it up and made a poultice from some of it, with which he bandaged the dog's leg. The poultice was replaced every few hours, and the dog made a complete recovery.[40] Despite its efficacy, the puffball has not been thoroughly investigated.[41]

Another common domestic emergency from earliest days must have been burns. Again, the list of known home remedies for burns consists of simple plant remedies, usually involving only one species, and that a native, easily-available one. Ivy leaves have been used right up to the twentieth century,[42] as have primrose

(*Primula vulgaris*) leaves.[43] Onion, cut and applied, is another widespread remedy for minor burns.[44] If we take the trouble to try to find out what these simple home remedies actually were, we discover not a web of myth and superstition but a list of home simples, some of which would have proved effective, and at least represented the best that was available.

Superstition, myth and magic seem to have developed not around self-medication but around any form of medication that involved the use of a healer. This can be amply illustrated from stories of healers that have come down to us in the written records. Ironically, these people, though relatively few in number, are better recorded in the literature than are the ordinary everyday people and their ordinary everyday cures. If it were not for the fact that many simple home remedies passed on orally have survived into the modern era, then we would probably remain in complete ignorance of what the vast majority of country people used for themselves as first-aid plant remedies. Simply because it is commonplace, and belongs to the lives of uneducated people, such information was rarely thought worth recording, even by early folklorists, who preferred the bizarre and spectacular. After all, the latter makes a better story!

In my opinion, the nineteenth-century folklorist Black actually turned the truth on its head when he claimed: 'In many cases the herb was only the accompaniment of magical words. There may have been merit in the plant in this case, or there may not have been. It was not necessary that it should have healing virtues; its merit lay in its emphasizing the charm.'[45] Now while this may have been true of the practice of healers, it emphatically was untrue of the simple plant remedies in everyday use. Unfortunately, Black lumps together under the heading of folk medicine both the plant remedies used on themselves by country people and the weird and wonderful remedies recorded as folk medicine in the literature. Approaching the subject from the premise that all folk medicine was based on superstition and magical practice, he interprets even practical instructions surrounding a remedy as evidence of superstition. For example, he quotes from the tenth- and eleventh-century *Herbarium Apuleii*, telling us that vervain (*Verbena officinalis*) is recommended for 'sore of liver', *if* taken on Midsummer day, and lithewort (*Sambucus ebulus*) for another complaint, *if* taken before the rising of the sun, 'in the month which is named July'[46] (my italics).

Just by the insertion of these two 'if's, the text becomes falsified. What were probably practical instructions as to the optimum time of day and year to gather the herbs become, in Black's hands, evidence of strange and supernatural superstitions. Grieve, in her *Modern Herbal*,[47] tells us that vervain 'must be picked before flowering and dried quickly'. And when does vervain flower? From July to September. In the *Herbarium Apuleii*, there are seven uses given for vervain, including: 'for sore of liver, take on Midsummer's day the same wort, and rub it to dust; take then five spoons full of the dust and three draughts of good wine; mix together; give to drink; it will benefit much'.[48] This reads like practical advice, rather than superstitious fantasy.

Here are the instructions for taking lithewort in the *Herbarium Apuleii*:

This wort, which is named hostriago, and by another name lithewort, is produced about burial places and on barrows, and on walls of houses, which stand against downs.

For all things which are generated on a man by way of disease, take this wort, which we called hostriago, and

knock (pound) it; then lay it to the sore. All things as we
ere said, which are generated on mans body to loathe, it
thoroughly will heal.

If thou will to take this wort, thou shalt be clean, and
also, ere rising of sun, thou shalt take it in the month
which is named July.[49]

Lithewort is identified as *Sambucus ebulus*, the dwarf elder,
which flowers from July to September. Again, these might
be practical instructions, rather than evidence of
superstitious practice. As mentioned in Chapter 2, the
identification in modern botanical terms of plants
mentioned in early written records is fraught with
difficulty. However, whatever the exact identification of
lithewort, the argument remains the same. Remedies
were often accompanied by practical instructions for
gathering the plant.

It does not seem too bold a claim to suggest that, from
earliest times, people discovered the healing as well as
edible properties of certain plants, and that such
knowledge would be handed down through the
generations, quite independently of the written word.
Once written records were kept, such knowledge would
feed into the corpus of official medical knowledge, and
doubtless this was at least to some extent a two-way
process, 'domestic' remedies being added to from written
and printed sources. On the whole, though, the traffic was
one-way, from traditional into official medicine. One has
only to look carefully at any of the mediaeval herbals to
see how many remedies are 'hearsay' from individuals.
Gerard, in his famous *Herbal*, quotes numerous incidents
of remedies learnt from ordinary individuals.[50]

Riddle has pointed out that 'many new early medieval
recipes are derived from folk medicine – Germanic, Celtic,
Hispanic and the like.'[51] A specific example of incorpora-

tion of a traditional remedy into orthodox practice is quoted by Nagy. In 1636 John Symcotts MD treated puerpera in one of his patients with a broth made from shepherd's purse. This he had learned from a beggar-woman. Presumably he was impressed with the results, since he continued to use it.[52]

All this would suggest that, alongside the development of official healing arts, the ordinary person continued to use tried and tested remedies, and sometimes to discover new ones. As Riddle puts it:

> Thousands, nay hundreds of thousands, of experiments in folk practice had separated those substances with pharmacological action from the inert and the harmful ... When one particular part of a herb, say a root, was found as being effective for some specific action, this information was orally transmitted whenever and wherever men communicated and one generation taught the other. This process takes place independently of literary transmission ... the writers are merely recording knowledge gained by folkways.[53]

It could be argued that the practical knowledge of plants as food and medicine pre-dates their use in magic, superstition and ritual. Stuart has called the hunter-gatherer period of human history, 'the longest clinical trial in history which eventually produced the herbs that provided the best foods, the poison to destroy enemies, the finest fuels and weapons, soporific drinks, medicines, the plants that produced colour for body and cave paintings, and the "magic" plants which carried primitive man away from reality.'[54]

Singer points out that there are remarkably few Palaeolithic drawings of plants, even though there are numerous surviving portraits of animals:

The reason for this neglect may be sought in the artist's motive. It is believed that these paintings were of a magical character; by representing the forms of animals on the walls of his cave the hunter thought to bring the animals within his power. The plant, since it needed no hunting, was neglected by the artist.[55]

Could the very familiarity of the plants used by people in food and medicine account for this neglect in the art of the Palaeolithic era, and in the art of the ancient Egyptians as well as the Greeks? Singer attributes this neglect of the plant in art to an anthropocentric attitude. However, one could argue that there was no reason to illustrate the well-known background of people's daily life. Only when a system of medicine began to develop would such illustrations be needed, to accompany learned instructions.

Discussing the numerous inaccuracies in plant identification that have taken place in written and printed sources, Singer also points out that it was not until the nineteenth century that natural history was taught in schools.[56] But this does not mean that the average person remained in ignorance about the plants he or she was surrounded by. Plants that were important, as food or medicine, would certainly have been recognized by people, and presumably described by their country names. The fact that confusion reigned in the pre-Linnaean era surrounding the *written* and *illustrated* identification of plants does not mean that the country people could not recognize accurately the native plants of their countryside, and in particular those plants that were important as food or medicine. Indeed, at least some of the local names for plants served as mnemonics for their use.

A twentieth-century example of this is the fact that in Norfolk, the field poppy remained known in some areas as the 'Headache' flower. One folklorist refers to this in the following patronizing manner: 'Wild Poppies are called "headaches" and are never brought into houses; they are considered to bring ill-luck to the gatherer.'[57] Here the written word seems to have distorted the truth. In fact, as discussed in Chapter 2, the field poppy has been used within living memory to *treat* headaches, especially those caused by a hangover.[58]

There are innumerable examples of local names for British plants that indicate their effects on man, e.g. 'piss-a-bed' for dandelion (*Taraxacum officinale*); 'bastard killer' for *Juniperus sabinus*, pilewort for *Ranunculus ficaria*. The list could be extended almost indefinitely. It is my opinion that some at least of the local names have been preserved orally, rather than in the literature, in much the same way that the remedies made from them have been preserved. Obviously, some local names are simply English translations or corruptions of the Linnaean Latin name, e.g. the Lanarkshire name 'dishyluggs' for coltsfoot (*Tussilago farfara*), but in many other instances they may pre-date the Linnaean name by many centuries. A startling example of this continuity of a local name is 'hayriffe', a gypsy name for *Galium aparine*, which is still used in Essex. In a thirteenth-century Anglo-Irish manuscript described by Tony Hunt, there is a remedy using the juice of 'heyreve' or 'heyrive', identified by Hunt as *Galium aparine*.[59]

Despite the manifest difficulties of identifying in modern terms the plants described in early literature, it is nevertheless possible to glean from written sources such as Riddle's some very valuable information concerning plant remedies. In his book, *Contraception and Abortion from the Ancient World to the Renaissance*, Riddle stresses the importance of oral transmission of knowledge concerning plants and fertility:

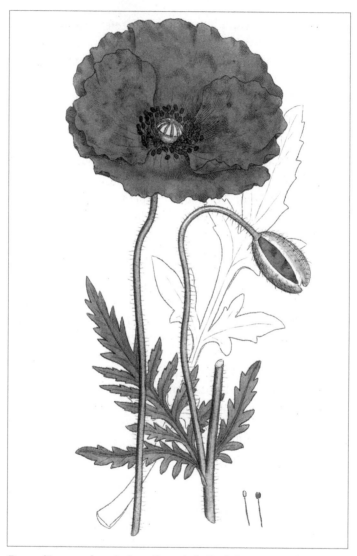

Poppy (*Papaver rhoeas*), from Sowerby's *English Botany.* (Photograph courtesy of John Innes Foundation Historical Collections)

The working knowledge of fertility plants was likely held by women and transmitted orally. Men, who wrote on the subject, were dependent on women as well as on their written sources ... From the British Isles to the eastern Mediterranean, late antiquity and the early Middle Ages knew about antifertility measures both from classical texts and from their own contributors. The question still becomes, how much did the common folk know, and how did they use what they knew? These questions are easy to pose, but so difficult to answer.[60]

Elsewhere in this same book,[61] writing about the Renaissance period, Riddle has some vivid examples of the link between 'folk' food and medicine:

Many of the antifertility plants fall into the category of pot herbs, the mints (e.g. pennyroyal, dittany (*Lepidium latifolium*) and sage (*Salvia officinalis*)) and rue, were served in salads or placed on meat. The woman's salad may have been her control over her life and her family's life, while the men and non childbearing women ate from the same bowl and saw it simply as a nourishing, tasty meal course. Rural people in India cook the roots of *Echinops echinatus* as part of their diet put there to control fertility. And control fertility it does, according to a 1988 laboratory study that found that the plant had 'very significant anti-oestrogenic activity'. The table use of this root in India parallels how Gargilius Martialis had said that women eat rue with their meals and do not have children. [Martialis was a retired soldier, writing in Africa in the third century AD.]

By and large, a person learned the information as orally transmitted lore, just as one would learn recipes for cooking. The cookbooks of the Middle Ages recorded vague instructions. The only practical way for the information to be learned was through experimentation.

It does seem highly likely that early plant medicine, wherever it was practised by ordinary people, was primarily an empirical use of the plants available. The difficulties of plant identification were probably compounded by the written word, not eased by it. The botanical Materia Medica for the ordinary people, anywhere in space or time, would be those plants readily available to them, in other words their own familiar native flora. However, once written records began, the problems of identification inevitably arose. One authority copied from another, and the practitioner, who relied on written information, would have to use whichever plant he thought approximated to the one in the written record. One could even argue therefore that the written record of plant medicine was *more* not less susceptible to error than the orally transmitted (and necessarily local) knowledge.

The infamous so-called doctrine of signatures, which flourished in the literature during the sixteenth and seventeenth centuries, is often quoted to illustrate the ignorance of country people in their use of plants. But, as we have seen in Chapter 1, this doctrine was invented, not by the primary users of plant remedies, but by Paracelsus, himself a man of learning and religion. According to this so-called doctrine, God set his seal on every plant, so that we might read it and see for what human purpose it will be useful. Thus the spotted leaves of the lungwort (*Pulmonaria officinalis*) plant indicate its use in lung complaints, the bulbous swellings on the lesser celandine (*Ranunculus ficaria*) roots indicate their usefulness in healing piles. Was the sixteenth- and seventeenth-century country-dweller really this gullible? I think not. It seems far more likely that the doctrine of signatures, as stated by Paracelsus, is a curious inversion of what was really a system of mnemonics in a society that depended heavily on memory and oral preservation of traditions.[62]

Thus, if the barberry plant was useful for liver complaints, it would be natural to seek a feature of the plant by which to remember this. The bright yellow bark could be associated with jaundice, so this would be a useful mnemonic. This seems to me a far likelier explanation.

Several exponents of the doctrine of signatures became quite carried away with it. By extension, all plants with yellow flowers could be supposed to be useful for jaundice. It is quite possible that in this way a large number of entirely specious plant remedies have crept into the literature, and Paracelsus may have done us all a great disservice. It would be of great interest to try to separate out these specious plant remedies, and to ascertain whether they are in fact among the least effective of the plant remedies recorded in the literature.

We have seen in earlier chapters how information fed into written literature from folk medicine, and, to a much lesser extent, flowed also from literature into folk medicine. During the Middle Ages, another custodian of knowledge was provided by the monasteries, and their manuscripts. While these drew heavily on medical literature of the day, they also undoubtedly incorporated a certain amount of 'folk' knowledge. Indeed, they were probably responsible for preserving some important knowledge which, rejected by the medical profession, might not otherwise have survived. In the murky area of abortion and contraception, about which many medical writers were afraid to give advice, monastic writings were sometimes less inhibited. The distinction between abortifacients and plants that brought on menstruation was a difficult and a dangerous one to make, and undoubtedly many abortions were brought about under the umbrella of correcting delayed menstruation.

Abortion has been and remains a highly emotive and controversial issue. However, folk knowledge of plants that brought about abortion was probably always greater than we realize. Even the common names of some of our British plants indicate that not all our forebears were so delicate in their dealings with such matters, as is shown by the Somerset name of 'bastard killer' for juniper. Since the time of Pliny, juniper (of various species) has been used as an abortifacient, and John Pechey in his seventeenth-century herbal was obviously well aware of the widespread unofficial use of the plant: 'It forces the courses and causes Miscarriage: Upon which account they are too well known and too much used by wenches.'[63]

Riddle points out that, when the medical literature began to drop official mention of plants that brought about abortion, such knowledge was preserved in some monastic writings. It may be that the plants of *Aristolochia*, which until recently grew in profusion in the grounds of the ruined Carrow Abbey in Norwich,[64] were used not just to ease the pains of childbirth, but also to procure abortions.

Ironically, too, warnings about the use of a particular herb in pregnancy are another way in which knowledge of abortifacients survived. The following extract is taken from a seventeenth-century manuscript:

To cause a woman to have her flowers

Tak of gladwin roots about a handfull. boyle them in vinegar or in white wine till they be very tender, and after put this into a vessell on the ground in a closse stooll so that the woman may sit over it – very close stopped so that the heat may strick up into her body – this medicine is reported never to faill but to bring them down. but you must have a speciall care that no woman being with childe have this medicine adminstered to her.[65]

Gladwin is probably a species of iris, most likely to be *Iris foetidissima*, which is still known by this name.

Another way in which religion influenced the development of traditional medicine was, of course, by the incorporation of prayers into the rituals used by healers. Because they are often bizarre and spectacular, much has been made in the literature of the so-called charms recorded in books of healing. It seems important again to stress the distinction between what was written down and what was actually used in practice by ordinary men and women. If a labourer cut his finger – whether with a flint or a ploughshare – it seems to me

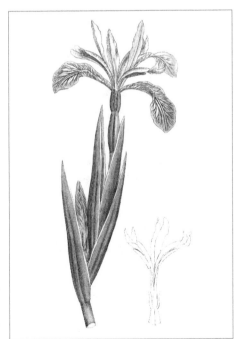

Gladden, stinking iris (*Iris foetidissima*), from Sowerby's *English Botany*. (Photograph courtesy of John Innes Foundation Historical Collections)

extraordinarily unlikely that he would use an elaborate charm to accompany the leaf or cobweb he used to bind it with. It is when an actual healer, whether religious, medical or simply a quack, steps in to treat illness that the charms and rituals develop. Given that, well into the eighteenth century, a high proportion of the users of domestic plant medicine in Britain were illiterate, the development of elaborate healing rituals may well have largely passed them by. This is not to suggest that religion played no part in their attempts to heal themselves. It would seem natural for a believer to back up the efficacy of a plant remedy with a prayer. One could even argue that the less effective the remedy, the more the need for prayer and other ceremony. A good example of this is a twentieth-century East Anglian home remedy for rheumatism: 'Boil the outside leaves of a cabbage in water till tender then strain. Drink half a cup of this each day. A sure cure for rheumatism – WITH FAITH.'[66]

In the face of incurable illness, it is worthwhile backing as many horses as possible! If this argument is carried to its logical conclusion, then one would expect the simple (and at least in some cases effective) plant remedies, used for relatively minor complaints, to be largely devoid of ceremony and superstition. This in fact appears to be the case. The hallmarks of a plant remedy that was actually used as self-medication are cheapness, ready availability, and lack of ceremony surrounding the remedy. This is the type of plant remedy that was passed down from one generation to the next by oral tradition.

Another scenario surrounds those plant remedies that were committed to writing, whether in early manuscripts or in printed books. These were subject to repetitive errors. Indeed, folklore in particular seems to be an area where authors copy and re-copy without question stories that in the first place may have been of doubtful accuracy. The misinterpretation of the name 'headache flower' in Chapter 2 is an example of this. Medical works on plant remedies were often copied from one century to the next, and from one country to another, and were moreover copied wholesale, with little reference to their effectiveness. Ironically, therefore, it is possible that the literature gives not only a false picture of domestic plant medicine, but actually an inverse picture, compared with those remedies actually in use.

Writing in 1694, the physician John Pechey, in his *Compleat Herbal*, says, 'I have only describ'd such Plants as grow in England, and are not commonly known; for I thought it needless to trouble the Reader with the Description of those that every Woman knows, or keeps in her Garden.'[67] What is *unwritten*, therefore, is the body of common knowledge surrounding common native British plants, but – as noted by many workers in the field of oral history – oral traditions are often preserved with remarkable accuracy, at least as long as they are in regular use.[68]

Because the written records give a false picture of the common use by ordinary people of familiar plants, present-day studies of oral history of plant medicine need to be recorded before this knowledge dies with the generation of elderly people who remember them. Such knowledge is usually taken for granted as a common practice, rather than seen as a valuable and interesting subject. Ask elderly country persons if they know anything about plant medicines, and they will probably deny any knowledge. Ask what their parents did for them when they were ill, and you might well elicit information, taken entirely for granted, concerning the use of plants for treating illness.

Trying to reconstruct our forebears' knowledge of plant medicine from present-day memories is like the field walker's task in archaeology. The whole has to be reconstructed from the shards remaining. The resultant picture is bound to be incomplete, and even inaccurate, but it is the best we can do. These remaining shards of knowledge have a special value in that they are vestiges of a knowledge of plant medicines selected by generations, and therefore they are likely to represent the most effective of the native plant remedies available. The wisdom of generations has creamed off the best of home remedies, and it would be a great and irreplaceable loss to ignore this knowledge.

Generally, domestic plant remedies were used in this country as simple first-aid measures, largely devoid of ritual or superstition. However, if we consider the subject of warts, this argument falters. An amazingly weird and wonderful collection of 'wart-cures' was the result of a recent Folklore Society Survey on the subject.[69] So strange and diverse are the methods used in this country for treating warts, that as one corespondent pointed out, they need a book to themselves. Now they are going to have at least a chapter![70] Despite most of the wart treatments being non-botanical, and therefore outside the scope of this book, a small selection of the methods used is presented in Chapter 6. The lack of botanical treatments in itself is of interest, tending to confirm that on the whole plant remedies were sensible and down-to-earth.

Allowing for warts as an exceptional case, the vast majority of domestic plant remedies used in Britain were probably empirical and largely devoid of either ritual or superstition. It is only when the treatment is no longer *self*-treatment, when a healer intervenes, that there is a likelihood of the remedies becoming clothed in ritual and obscurity. This development is a two-way one. The sufferer casts himself in the role of 'patient', and expects more from his healer than the home remedies with which he is already familiar. The healer responds by developing a 'system' of healing that erects a barrier between patient and healer, one that is reinforced by the patient's wish to see the healer as in some way superior, or at least as having superior knowledge. The healer may obscure remedies by surrounding them with ritual, or by using a language (such as Latin) unfamiliar to the patient, and this can be said of both official and unofficial healers in medicine.

4

THE PEOPLE THEMSELVES

The Users of Domestic Medicine

Domestic plant medicine was a necessity of daily life during the last three centuries. Its practitioners, ordinary country-dwellers, either lacked access to orthodox medicine or could not afford it. The reasons for the decline in the use of plant medicine can be summarized briefly as an increase in availability of orthodox medicine, improved transport from the countryside into the towns, and a reduction in the number of agricultural workers with increased mechanization and increased farm size.

The 'typical' user of domestic plant medicines at the beginning of the twentieth century was probably the agricultural labourer and his family, for whom it provided cheap first aid. Just how hard life was in those days most of us probably cannot appreciate. Mr G. was born in Norfolk in 1900. He was one of five children, his mother died of consumption when he was three and, in his own understated words, 'food was difficult'. His father managed as best he could; sometimes he got a free bullock's head from the butcher, which, stewed with carrots, turnips and onions, would last them all a week.

The only first aid he remembered was a raw onion, rubbed on a burn to take the pain out.[1]

A similarly harsh life is portrayed by Mrs Vera W., brought up on the Halvergate marshes by her grandmother in the early years of the twentieth century. Granny used cobwebs for bad cuts, but for minor ones, you had to 'swish your hand around in a pail of cold water until the water was all red, then bind it up and leave it bound for a week'. As a little girl, Vera remembers going in the pony and trap to Great Yarmouth on market day. Granny always wore her black cloak, and when they reached the toll, Vera had to hide inside the cloak to avoid paying the halfpenny![2] For abscesses, a poultice was made from houseleek (*Sempervivum tectorum*). This plant figures repeatedly in rural first aid, and was often encouraged to grow on the roofs of outbuildings.

Mrs D. was born at Reedham in 1902. She was one of fourteen, seven girls and seven boys. Her mother made bread on Tuesdays and Fridays, and on these days her father got up extra early to light the fire to warm the bread oven. She remembers as a treat the occasions when they had bread rolls, split open, with a little lump of cheese inside; the roll was then popped back in the oven for a few minutes. They were delicious! She says that the children were rarely ill, and attributes this to the fact that their food was plain but healthy. First aid consisted of a mustard plaster on the chest for a cold, salt for toothache, and a roasted onion warmed and placed inside the ear for earache.[3] In another Norfolk family, roasted shallot took the place of onion for earache.[4] Onions were frequently used to treat minor burns.

Another readily available Norfolk plant was used by Mrs J., of Salhouse; the leaves of alder (*Alnus glutinosa*) were used by her family to treat burns.[5] The same lady recollects a large fig tree that grew in the garden. Its leaves were used to treat warts. Another lady from Cambridgeshire remembers the 'Heal-All' tree that grew in her childhood garden. The leaves were used to treat infected wounds; the upper, smooth side to 'draw' the puss, the lower to heal it. The identity of this plant is uncertain; it may have been roseroot (*Sedum rosea*).

Numerous people recollect using puffballs to stop bleeding, in both animals and humans. One elderly Norfolk man recalls that his grandfather always kept a 'bulfer' (puffball, *Lycoperdon* sp.) hanging in the garden shed for use in emergencies.[6] A similar use is described by a Suffolk lady, now in her seventies, whose dog was rescued after an accident in which an artery in its leg was torn (see p. 131). Her uncle fetched a large 'Smoky Jo' and showed her how to make a poultice. The leg healed cleanly.[7]

Horseradish root (*Armoracia rusticana*)was sometimes used to heal cuts, as well as for treating sore throats.[8] There is a particularly vivid account from a woman living in Yorkshire who had a serious cut on her leg:

My grandfather was a great believer in herbal medicine, I regret deeply not showing more interest in what he did. He could neither read nor write, but he would collect his remedies and put them in strong white bags, and hang them on a beam in the bedroom, each bag had a mark telling what it contained, and only he knew what that was. When a child I cut my arm very badly in a V-shape that looked like a pig's mouth. My granddad told an aunt to 'get a clean clart' he dug up a campher root scrubbed it clean, grated it on to the cloth and bound it tight round my arm. As the cloth dried and tightened on my arm I had to keep wetting the cloth with cold water. The cut healed quickly and the scar is very tiny it's hard to imagine the cut was so big, and deep. I am now 73, my granddad died

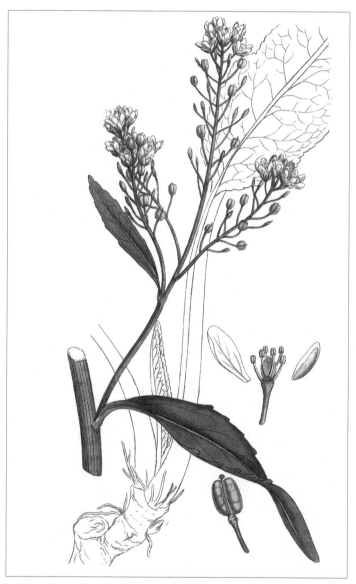

Horseradish (*Armoracia rusticana*), from Sowerby's *English Botany*.
(Photograph courtesy of John Innes Foundation Historical Collections)

of old age at 88 he kept most of the family well with his knowledge.[9]

The identity of the 'campher' plant is unclear. It could be *Crithmum maritimum*, which is known as 'Camphire' in Cumberland,[10] but this seems unlikely, the root being hardly suitable for grating. Perhaps it was horse-radish (*Armoracia rusticana*), used to treat cuts, sore throats and neuralgia in East Anglia? We may never know the identity of the plant used; this is one of very numerous examples where the detailed knowledge of plant use has been forgotten.

A vivid account of a now-forgotten use of foxglove leaves (*Digitalis purpurea*) comes from an elderly lady whose childhood was spent in Wales:

My mother had eleven children and I was the eldest girl ... Mother breast fed all of us and when she weaned the baby we went into the woods to gather the largest leaves of the Foxgloves. These she (mother) put on her breasts like plasters. They dried her milk with no ill effects. Another remedy I remember was the cure for all bumps, cuts and bruises, was the dock leaf, these too were applied to the wound like plasters, and stopped the bleeding and brought down the bump.

In those far off days we had many a cut and graze when playing in the hills.

We never had a doctor, coughs and colds in the winter, mother treated us to boiled onions thickened with cornflour and milk before going to bed. How it made me sweat. We have all, up till now, lived to a good healthy old age. The baby of the family is now 65. I was 86 last August, still keeping very well, on a simple diet ...

When I go out for a walk I look at the elder berries left to rot on the trees. They are really medicine, made into wine,

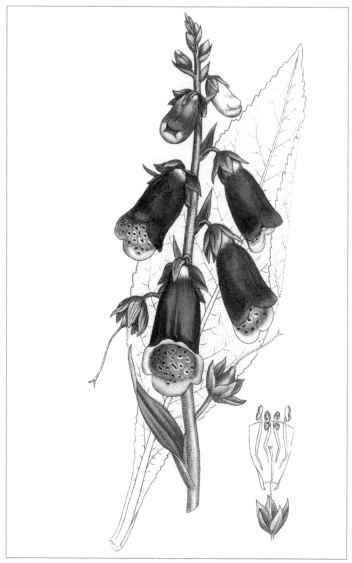

Foxglove (*Digitalis purpurea*), from Sowerby's *English Botany*.
(Photograph courtesy of John Innes Foundation Historical Collections)

nothing could beat a glass of elderberry wine. The cure-all for all ills, at least I think so.[11]

None of this knowledge was seen as specialized in any way by its users; it was simply part of life to use the plants on hand to treat ailments. A number of vivid descriptions by individuals knowledgeable about domestic herbal medicines are contained in a collection of essays written for a competition organized by Age Concern in Essex in 1990. The writers of these essays have preserved a glimpse of an otherwise under-recorded aspect of life in this country in the early years of the twentieth century:

Great-aunt Alice Flack was a real, old Essex lady: tall and stately yet down-to-earth and always ready for a chat ...

It must have been during these late-nineteenth century years in Rayleigh that Alice developed her knowledge of remedies and local 'cure-alls' that I remember her for. This would have been when most of the town's roads were unmade and the Weir was a pond. Long, ranging hedgerows and patchy scrub-land would have covered huge tracts of what are now housing estates. Here among the wild flowers and grasses she would have gathered various herbs in order to try a new cure, or relief, of some kind.

For a sore throat I remember her telling my mother to pour a pint of boiling water on to twenty-five sage leaves. Then, after half an hour, add a little vinegar and honey (according to taste). The resulting infusion to be gargled with three times a day. From memory I believe it had to be light on vinegar and heavy on honey to suit me!

On the occasions when my grandfather (her brother-in-law) complained of broken chilblains she would mix a large glass of flower-oil with three ounces of spirit of turpentine. Then with half a pound of pig's lard and three ounces of bee's wax she would stir the mixture over a slow fire until the wax was melted. Next day it would be ready for use and could be applied by smearing on the affected part with a soft cloth ...

The treatment of wasp, and particularly bee, stings was variously carried out by: hartshorn drops, sweet oil, juice of onion or washing-day blue-bag.

Stinging nettle rash could be soothed by rubbing with rosemary, mint or sage leaves. Dock leaves were also considered.

To remove freckles Alice advocated that an ounce of lemon juice, a quarter dramme of powdered borax and a dramme of sugar, mixed and left to stand for a few days in a bottle, would do the job ...

I don't know how effective some of Alice's cures were but I know that she was a popular woman and I suppose that would not have been the case if she'd been wrong too often.

What did used to impress me was her belief that for most ills there was a nearby remedy e.g. nettle and dock, marsh fever and willow (*Salix* spp.) aspirin.

Great Aunt Alice learnt many of her divers remedies from older relatives and friends but some were created by her own invention.[12]

Here are some more vivid recollections from an early twentieth-century rural childhood:

In this day and age we think nothing of going to the doctor for any troubles that might ail us and take our prescription to the chemist as a matter of course. We are used to do it and take it for granted, we hardly ever recall how it used to be. Years ago things were quite different and we had all to be a lot more self reliant as far as illnesses and remedies were concerned. The doctor's surgery was miles away and for minor ailments the elders of the community were consulted.

I grew up in a small village at the edge of a forest. The oldest little house consisted only of a small kitchen with a square brick fireplace in the centre for cooking and one large room for living and sleeping. Here lived the cooper with his wife. We children watched him going round in circles with two hammers driving hoops on to the wooden barrels which were used by the villagers for their home made scrumpy cider. The fresh apple juice from the press was nice and sweet and the best remedy for constipation.

During summer children walked without shoes and one day I had a rusty nail sticking in my foot. I pulled it out myself and carried on playing. After some days my foot became painful and I noticed pus coming from the wound. Granny went to the nearby woods and collected resin from the pine [*Pinus* sp.] trees. This was put on a little linen pad, softened on the kitchen range and put onto my sore. I soon could feel a drawing sensation. When checked after some days, the wound was beautifully clean and it had healed nicely.

When I had swollen legs from an insect bite, a linseed [*Linum usitatissimum*] poultice was made and put on my legs, which helped.[13]

Here is another insight into country life at the beginning of this century in Essex:

On Friday nights the children lined up for their dose of liquorice or brimstone and treacle, as Saturday they would be home for this to act, and mother was sure they would be alright for another week. I remember when I was small I was given the same medicine.

The winters used to be very cold in those days, so the children got chilblains on hands and feet. Mother made

them use the chamber pot, then they had to dip their hands
and feet in this which helped a lot and stopped the irritation.
I had to do the same and it did help as they did itch.[14]

In the family portrayed in the next extract, it was
grandmother who was the main authority on healing
plants:

During that period known as 'between the wars' when
many of today's pensioners were being brought up
without the benefit of the National Health system it was a
good time for those with money but a bad time for workers
who were badly paid or had no work in the General Strike
and no money for doctor's bills. People had their own
cures. Many handed down from mediaeval times.

We were lucky enough to live in the country and to have
a grandmother who understood the healing powers of
plants. 'All plants are useful', she would say 'Only their
misuse is evil.' 'Ee-law' leaves were used on one side for
healing and on the other side for drawing such as boils or
whitlows although whitlows had their own cures in
whitlow grass or whitlow wort. Ee-law, I discovered
eventually, should have been Heal-All. Probably a variety
of Valerian.

Winter, as always was a trying time and it was not
unknown for the Victorian child, if inclined to be 'chesty'
to have its little body rubbed with goose fat and sewed into
a flannel vest not to be removed until May was out. The old
adage 'Ne'er cast a clout till May be out' left in doubt
whether the May referred to was the month or the blossom
(hawthorne). Feet itching from painful chilblains could be
thrust into a chamber pot while the sufferer's urine was
still warm or alternatively rubbed with raw onion ...

Great emphasis was placed on keeping the bowels open
and the pores closed and on cleansing the blood after the

rigours of winter and so, in the spring we were sent to gather young nettles. We also gathered elderflowers (and elderberries for wine) which was used in so many remedies, with a base of pure lard, elderflower water went into embrocations, ointments, salves and creams. It was also used as an astringent.

The doctor was called only for serious illnesses when a coal fire was lit in the bedroom and the patient nursed night and day until he or she passed the 'crisis'. I remember straw being spread on the road outside the houses of sick people to deaden the sound of cars, horses or horse-drawn vehicles until that moment of crisis was past and they could be given beef tea and arrowroot to help them regain their strength ...

When I had whooping cough I was fed a concoction of cod liver oil, glycerine, lemon juice, soft brown sugar, finely chopped onion, black treacle, ground ginger, cinnamon and vinegar. I may have left out a few items but still remember the taste ...

Our grandmother wearing what must have been the last of the proper sunbonnets (I have never seen another) gathered goosegrass which she cooked and fed to the goslings, hence the name, but a pad soaked in the liquid and bandaged over a wound was supposed to help the tissue to knit quickly. Goosegrass is the weed that children call Sweethearts probably because of its propensity to cling. We were not asked to gather it as the seeds were too tiresome to remove from our clothing. Enough said![15]

These vivid glimpses of rural life in the early years of the century provide an insight into the type of people who used do-it-yourself plant medicines out of tradition and out of necessity. In contrast, the city dweller could not go out into the hedgerows to gather herbs. Not surprisingly, we find that the urban practitioner of home remedies used a different pharmacopoeia, relying on garden plants and on dried herbs from the chemist, as well as home remedies not of plant origin. The following account illustrates the uses of urban home remedies:

Years ago money was very scarce we had to find remedies for ourselfs.

My mother used to make us brown paper vests to put on next to our skin to save the cold winds getting to our chest.

My Dad used to work in Smithfield meat market, and every Christmas he was given a goose. When mother had cooked the goose the fat from it she used to put on the brown paper on our chest. This was a good remedy. And if we had a high temperature she would keep us in bed for about three days and boil some onions and milk to give us, she never worried if we did not eat as long as we had plenty to drink.

If we had a sore throat she would put a silk stocking round our neck, and make us gargle with salt water, as we got older we used to use camphorated oil on our chest.

When you had a family you could not keep having a Doctor home at three shillings and sixpence, that was a lot of money out of a weekly wage.

When we went to school we had boots that buttoned up at the side with a button hook, and mother would wrap newspaper round our feet before we put our boots on so our feet would not get cold in winter.

Whenever we had earache we used to get a poppy seed head from the chemist (twopence) and mother used to bind that round our ear.

If we had a splinter or a whitlow and it started festering mother would make a poultice of sunlight soap and sugar that used to do the trick.

Every Friday night was bath night and after we had it we used to have a dose of Epsom salts and a sulphur tablet.

When we were little, mother used to say sweets rot your teeth so we would go to the greengrocer and buy halfpenny of specks (they were not specks) but when the apples and oranges got bruised the greengrocer would cut the bad away and give us the good, we used to get a lot for a halfpenny, a carrot thrown in, we used to love going to school chewing them. I think they were good old days, we didn't have much money but we were happy and healthy.[16]

In the cities as in the countryside, in addition to family members who prepared home remedies, there were sometimes local experts to turn to for advice:

I was born in 1920 and spent my childhood in a mining village, the rows of terraced houses facing each other across cobbled streets. Every neighbour knew each other, shared their troubles, their happiness, their sickness. Illness was consulted, decided, and often treated without calling in the local GP.

The 'Head Consultant' lived at Number 73, a white-haired, long, white bearded old man by the name of Christmas Davis – Yes, that was his real name, children held him in awe and I can visualise him now sat in a Wooden arm chair always smoking a Clay pipe. He had a Philosophy that there was a Herb for every illness known to mankind. All mothers-to-be were prescribed an infusion of Raspberry tea, taken throughout their pregnancy, for an easy delivery.

Parsley Tea for Bladder troubles; Thyme for indigestion and Stomach Acidity, Wormwood tea for a Tonic, and Depression. Sage tea for the menopause. Camomile tea for headaches.

The strange thing was that very often the Herb prescribed perhaps for falling hair was often the same as for some other ailment. No matter of argument, the afflicted had faith in these remedies, believed in them and found relief in their usage.

I think I saw the start of alternative Medicine in those early days!

My Grandmother was more orthodox, and often drastic in her treatments, one dare hardly complain of any malady as her cures were often more painful than the disease. If one complained of Ear-ache a Poultice of Boiled Onions was secured to the offending ear and fastened round the head with a long white strip of cotton material-Turban-style one walked about like an Egyptian Mummy. If this did not produce the desired effect it was taken off and a few drops of olive oil was put in the ear, completed with a plug of cotton wool for drainage. Boils were destined to plasters of White Windsor soap grated and mixed with sugar: a painful procedure when they had to be peeled off!

Her own frequent headaches always had the same remedy – a little grated Nutmeg in warm water.

Sore, or inflamed eyes were often relieved by a few drops of Castor Oil. This did prove effective.

Friday night was always set apart for the weekly dose of Brimstone and Treacle or an infusion of Senna pods, to 'clear the system out'.

My grandfather often suffered the humiliation of having the lower part of his back covered in brown paper and ironed briskly with the flat iron to relieve his lumbago: a sure cure if the iron became too hot!

The common cold was always regarded with reverence, and grave doubts. 'It can turn into Pneumonia' was always the premonition, so it was always the same advice, and treatment. Packed off to bed with hot water bottle and extra blankets. Hot milk, with the butcher's suet shredded, and a little sugar added, a Beecham's powder and if you complained of a Sore Throat your woollen sock (the sweatier the better!) was fastened loosely round your neck. The chest rubbed liberally with camphorated oil, should you be well enough to attend school next day, the sock was replaced by a band of flannel secured by a large safety pin. If a cough developed Grandma would roast a number of turnips, press the juice out of them, add a little sugar and subject the victim to three Wine glassfuls a day. A cold didn't stand a chance!!

Maybe these remedies seem old fashioned today and yet I still remember them with deep affection. I had to see the doctor today with a Sore Throat, he prescribed antibiotics ... but as an extra precaution I think I will wrap my stocking loosely round my neck at Bed time.

I doubt if Grannie would approve. Tights may not have the same Medicinal value as an old woollen sock.[17]

The subject of domestic 'chemist' remedies, used by town and, to a lesser extent, by country people is an interesting aspect of domestic medicine that really requires a book to itself. In the present volume, we are mainly concerned with domestic plant remedies.

If we assume a broad basis of common knowledge of plant remedies among country dwellers, then there would have been little need for any specialized practitioners; it was everybody's province. But it is in the nature of human communities to produce 'experts' in almost everything, and plant medicines were no exception. As no record of domestic plant medicine would be complete without this specialist knowledge, in my research I endeavoured to include accounts by these practitioners. For the researcher, it is tantalizing how often one comes across glimpses of individuals who used plant medicines, but are now largely forgotten, even by members of their own family. As young children, we are rarely interested in the knowledge of our grandparents, and when such knowledge is no longer in practical daily use, it quickly becomes lost. I have frequently been told about individuals who 'knew cures for everything', but in many cases, the informant cannot remember which plant was used for which remedy.

In Rockland St Mary in the early years of the twentieth century there lived two sisters who were often to be seen gathering plants in the hedgerows, and in their kitchen there was always a brew on the stove. Local children were evidently slightly afraid of these two old ladies, and did not like being sent by their mothers to fetch a herbal brew. The only remedies made by them that my informant remembered were coltsfoot wine, and 'pickacheese' poultices. (The latter, made from mallow shoots, were used for festered fingers and abscesses.)[18] Another East Anglian has vivid memories of an old lady who used to come to the house every springtime, with a concoction in which little green apples were bobbing about. This was given to the reluctant children as a springtime cleanser. The informant had no idea what was in the syrup![19]

A man now in his seventies related how, when he was a small child, his whole family were ill with flu, and a local expert was called in, an old lady who dosed them with a 'very powerful' brew, containing onions and other ingredients that he could not recall. It tasted dreadful, but it soon got them all back on their feet.[20]

An elderly relative was sometimes the family expert on plant remedies. Mrs A., now living in Norfolk, recalls as a child in Dovercourt, Essex, being sent by her granny to gather sea lettuce in a screw-top jar. She had to fill up the jar with sea water. Granny heated up both on the stove, and the seaweed was slapped on to relieve the pain of bunions. The water was used as a foot-bath to relieve sore feet. Granny was of Irish extraction; other remedies recalled by her grand-daughter include an infusion of lime (*Tilia* (x *cordata*)) flowers to cure headache, and houseleek juice to keep the skin clear. Granny's ointment for cuts and grazes, made from yarrow (*Achillea millefolium*) was locally famous, and each year a large batch was made up for family use and for friends and neighbours.[21]

Mrs H. now lives alone in a small remote cottage on a common in Norfolk. She inherited the cottage from her aunt, who apparently knew the names of all the innumerable different plants on the common. Mrs H. remembers a few of her aunt's remedies, including an infusion of vervain leaves for sunburn. The water in which young nettle tops have been boiled is used by Mrs H. for treating arthritis, and when friends have flu or a cold, she always recommends hot infusion of the wild

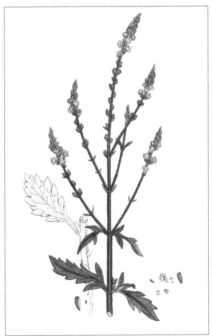

Vervain (*Verbena officinalis*), from Sowerby's *English Botany*. (Photograph courtesy of John Innes Foundation Historical Collections)

mint that grows on the marshes near her cottage. She said, though, that when she recently had flu it did not occur to her to use mint infusion, because 'when you have a remedy, you don't use it'! Mrs H. keeps ponies, chickens and geese. If they are under the weather, they are fed with the comfrey that she grows in her garden.

Another instance of someone brought up by a grandparent illustrates very vividly how swiftly oral traditions cross the centuries. Mr M, now in his seventies, was brought up his grandmother, Jeannie, in Ayrshire and later in Stirlingshire. Jeannie was born about 1880. She was always amazingly lucky in draws and raffles, so much so that sometimes she was asked not to enter them! She was evidently a stern woman, but clearly remembered with affection. The effectiveness of her remedies was acknowledged even by the local doctor. She used leeches from the stream for bad bruises: cow dung for bad legs ('that'll cure his leg, laddie'), cobwebs for deep cuts, salt for all kinds of things, including as a gargle. They had few fresh vegetables, but granny used to put all kinds of plants into the soup, including nettles, dandelion and fat hen. To this day, Mr M. still eats dock leaves, when he can get clean ones! Mr M. vividly remembers the time when one of his childhood friends was scalded on the face. Granny sent him to collect ivy leaves from the stable wall. Granny dressed the burnt face with ivy leaves, olive oil and vinegar, covered with a 'mask' with eye holes. The face healed without a blister.

When Jeannie was a child, her grandmother told her the story of a village in Ayrshire where a fever epidemic killed a large proportion of the population. One family hung a bag of onions on their door, and no one in that family became ill. This was so striking that the story has been handed down four generations. The epidemic in the Ayrshire village must have occurred in the early part of the nineteenth century, and was being related nearly two hundred years later. This is an example of the way in which the spoken word skims the centuries. Oral history can indeed take us back further in time than one might imagine.

In East Anglian villages, and probably also in other regions of the country, there was often a lady who acted as midwife and layer-out of the dead. She was sometimes an expert on home remedies: 'Long after more skilled medical help was available, the health of a family largely remained, especially in rural areas, the responsibility of the housewife, with or without the aid of that invaluable person, the local nurse-cum-midwife-cum-wise-woman.'[22] Frederick Wigby, author of *Just A Country Boy*,[23] gives this vivid description of the unofficial (and unpaid) midwife who brought him into the world at Wicklewood, Norfolk, in 1912:

Granny Davis was a wonderful old lady. The lady on the advert for 'Robinson's Starch' was exactly like her: when it used to be on the bill hoardings it always reminded me of her.

She brought most of the children in the village into the world and laid out those who had passed on. As there were no chapels of rest the corpse was placed in a coffin, placed on trestles, and left there until the funeral. In summertime Feverfew was placed around it and also on the lid as it was taken to the place of burial. Many seeds of the Feverfew fell off en route and that is why the plant is or was frequently found in many village churchyards, mainly on the north side where the paupers were buried, or those who had committed suicide.

Granny used the following plant remedies. Ground Ivy [*Glechoma hederacea*], with Celandine and Daisies crushed and strained, sugar and rose water were added to remove inflammation in the eyes. Wild Tansy [*Tanacetum vulgare*] rubbed on meat joints kept blow flies off it. Garden Poppy [*Papaver* spp.] petals macerated and mixed with milk in babies' bottles was used for fevers. Black Currant leaves rubbed on gums helped teething. Laudanum was freely available in those days, Granny used it quite a lot and regularly put a drop in babies' bottles, as did many a mother.

Here are a few of the old names that Granny used to call many plants and Herbs. Hearts-ease [*Viola* sp.] was known as Three-faces-in-one-hood; Trinity herb, Love-in-idleness. The Stonecrop [*Sedum acre*] went by the name of Welcome-Home-Husband-though-ever-so-drunk. The summer flowering Dracocephalum was called by many elderly folk Dragon's Head. Herb Bennet was the Avens; Herb Christopher for the Baneberries, Herb Gerarde for Goutweed, Herb Impious for the Cudweed, Herb Robert for the Cranesbill, Herb Two-pence for the Loosestrife.

Granny made a wonderful home made beer from hops, Horehound and malt which was in great demand in hot weather. For nursing mothers she made up a decoction of sifted bran, oats and skim milk, which, when boiled helped them to recover much quicker.[24]

Granny Davis used numerous other plant remedies too, which are described in Wigby's book.[25]

Where did practitioners such as Granny Davis obtain their information? Presumably they collected plant remedies in the course of their practice, but it is quite possible that at least some of their knowledge was gleaned from books. An analysis of Granny Davis' remedies shows that almost half of them bear a very strong resemblance to remedies to be found in Gerard's *Herbal*, so perhaps she was the owner of a copy of this book. The similarities can be seen clearly in the following comparison of remedies reported by Frederick Wigby with those of Gerard:

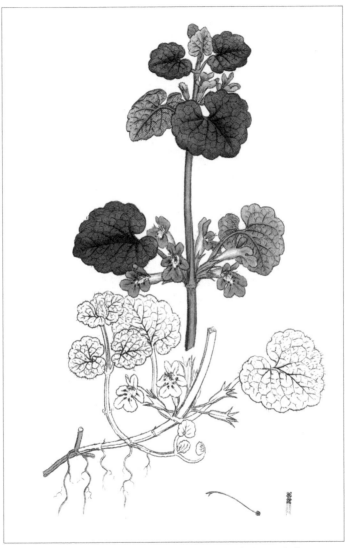

Ground Ivy (*Glechoma hederacea*), from Sowerby's *English Botany*.
(Photograph courtesy of John Innes Foundation Historical Collections)

Ground Ivy, with Celandine and Daisies crushed and strained, sugar and rose water were added to remove inflammation in the eyes.'[26]

Compare this with the following remedy described by Gerard:

Ground-Ivy, Celandine, and Daisies, of each a like quantitie, stamped and strained, and a little sugar and rose water put thereto, and dropped with a feather into the eies, taketh away all manner of inflammation, spots, webs, itch, smarting, or any griefe whatsoever in the eyes, yea although the sight were nigh hand gone: it is proved to be the best medicine in the world.[27]

In his book, Frederick Wigby tells us that:

Children having trouble teething were given groundsel softened in milk: this was supposed to soften the gums and make teething less sore.[28]

In Gerard we read, under the 'vertues' of Groundsel

The leaves stamped and strained into milke and drunke, helpe the red gums and frets in children.[29]

Granny Davis recommended Henbane (*Hyoscyamus niger*) root soaked in vinegar for toothache:[30]

Gerard, describing the virtues of Henbane, claims:

The root boiled with vinegre, & the same holden hot in the mouth, easeth the pain of the teeth.[31]

Granny Davis used:

A decoction from the green leaves or roots of Coltsfoot for coughs.[32]

Under the virtues of coltsfoot, Gerard gives:

A decoction made of the greene leaves and roots, or else a syrrup thereof, is good for the cough that proceedeth of a thin rheume.[33]

Granny Davis used:

Thorn-apple boiled in pork grease for inflammations, burns and scalds.[34]

In Gerard we read:

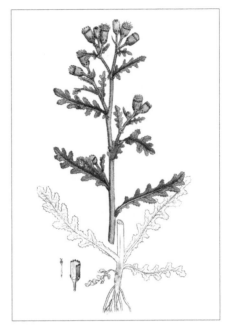

Groundsel (*Senecio vulgaris*), from Sowerby's *English Botany*. (Photograph courtesy of John Innes Foundation Historical Collections)

The juice of Thorn-apples boiled with hogs grease to the form of an unguent or salve, cures all inflammations whatsoever, all manner of burnings or scaldings, as well of fire, water, boiling lead, gun pouder, as that which comes by lightning, and that in very short time, as my selfe have found by my daily practise, to my great credit and profit. The first experience came from Colchester, where Mistress *Lobel* a merchants wife there being most grievously burned by lightning, and not finding ease or cure in any other thing, by this found helpe and was perfectly cured when all hope was past, by the report of Mr *William Ram* publique notarie of the same towne.[35]

Out of thirteen remedies described by Frederick Wigby as being used in the early years of the twentieth century by Granny Davis, five of them are clearly recognizable in

Gerard's *Herbal*, and may well have been derived from it. While one might have expected to find herbal practitioners drawing on Gerard and other printed herbals during the seventeenth century, it is at first sight surprising to find such a direct link in the twentieth century.

Agnes Arber describes a nineteenth-century practitioner who used Gerard's *Herbal* similarly:

> The present writer was once told by a man who was born in 1842 that, during his boyhood in Bedfordshire, he was acquainted with a cottager who treated the ailments of her neighbours with the help of a copy of Gerard's *Herbal*. If, as is most likely, this was one of Johnson's editions, she must thence have known certain illustrations copied from Anicia Juliana's manuscript of Dioscorides made soon after AD 500 – figures which were probably themselves derived from the work of Krateuas, belonging to the century before Christ. We thus catch a glimpse of the herbal tradition passing unbroken through two thousand years, from Krateuas, the Greek, to an old woman poring over her well-thumbed picture-book in an English village.[36]

Sadly, it is unusual to find any record of the actual plant remedies used by such local experts. Often the memories of other household remedies remain more vivid, such as the notorious goosegrease rubbed on a chest for a cold (see below), or the Friday night dose of brimstone and treacle (see p. 157). In the following extract we have a picture of a local unofficial midwife in Kent:

> Living as a child in the middle of the Romney Marsh in Kent, where the only means of transport were a bicycle or walking and the nearest doctor four-and-a-half miles away, each family had its own 'Patent Medicines'.

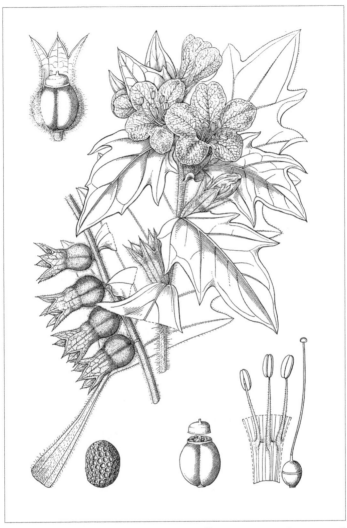

Henbane (*Hyoscyamus niger*), from Stella Ross-Craig, *Drawings of British Plants.* (By kind permission of the Royal Botanical Gardens, Kew/photograph courtesy of John Innes Foundation Historical Collections)

When we needed help, we naturally went to my Gran, who would not only cure us but was also the area midwife. She had helped to deliver over 250 babies before the law in 1936 said only registered midwives could deliver babies.

There was the usual remedy of goose grease rubbed on chest and back for a cold. (This sometimes smelt a bit but it seemed to do the trick.)

Vinegar too was widely used – not only was it rubbed on bruises but, after a sprain had been held first in hot water and then in cold, a bandage soaked in vinegar was applied.

I remember too mother adding some to the rinse water when washing our hair – not only to give it a shine but also to kill any 'creepy crawlies' we might have picked up at school. If we had a boil that took a while to burst or had a thorn or sliver of wood which needed to be 'drawn out', it was always cured with a bread poultice. This was made by putting a slice of bread between two pieces of cloth, covered with boiling water and wrung out. When I had a quinsey throat, I had one on the outside of my throat and another inside my mouth – it worked!

A 'Blue Bag', which was always used in the last rinse water to keep clothes white, was always used on wasp or bee stings but for a sting by nettles, there was nearly always a dock leaf growing nearby to stop the itch.

Other herbal cures were nettle tea, made by boiling the heads of stinging nettles, then straining and drinking the water. This was very tasty with sugar and was a very good cure for a rash.

A weed called Sun Spurge, which grew all over the Marsh, was used to cure warts. Inside the stem there is a milky fluid and, applied for about a week, would soon get rid of the warts.

My Gran also made an ointment by crushing the seeds of the Marsh Mallow plant and mixing it with pure lard.

This would soon help to heal a sore that was taking rather a long time to get better.[37]

First-hand information such as this is unfortunately rare. All too often 'Granny's remedies' are portrayed in present-day literature as the eccentric, useless and sometimes bizarre beliefs of an earlier age. In fact, they represent a body of common-sense first aid, built up over many centuries, and used as part of daily life.

Given the fragmentary nature of our information concerning twentieth-century domestic medicine in this country, it is hardly surprising to find that, as we go back in time, even less is known. Gervase Markham, writing during the seventeenth century, emphasizes medical knowledge as of paramount importance among essential womanly skills.[38] Unfortunately, details of such domestic medical knowledge rarely survive. As Porter has pointed out:

> The past is all too often silent: essential evidence simply has not survived. Thus it is highly probable that large numbers of female healers (so-called 'wise women') possessed valuable medical skills in traditional society ... Unfortunately, whereas a fair number of autobiographies and case-books of male practitioners survive, we lack equivalents from female healers. Their outlooks and practices must be deduced second or third hand, often from highly hostile sources.[39]

Those fragments of information that are available suggest that the world of domestic remedies, whether family ones or those used by local experts, was distinct from official herbalism, though there was obviously an overlap, and information could pass between the two, in both directions.

It is impossible to ascertain whether most local herbal 'experts' had book knowledge in addition to the common

body of orally transmitted information. One startling
example where this was true is to be found in the life of
Adam Donald, born in Bethelnie in Aberdeenshire in 1703.
He was the son of a cottar, and was born handicapped and
unfit for the work of a labourer. The account we have of
him was published in the eighteenth-century journal *The
Bee*, written by a lawyer, who clearly disliked the fame that
Adam acquired. His account, while biased, at least has the
virtue of being more or less contemporary:

Adam Donald ... was, for many years, known by no other
name than that of the prophet of Bethelnie ... His parents
were in no respect distinguished from the ordinary class of
poor people in that country, who, at that time, found great
difficulty to provide a scanty subsistence for themselves.
Nor could their son, from the distorted nature of his body,
undertake the fatigue of those robust employments in
which people, who live in the country, must engage for
obtaining their subsistence. He therefore was induced to
amuse himself with such books as chance enabled him to
obtain; and though he could scarcely read the English
language, yet he carefully picked up books in all languages
that fell in his way; and the writer has at present, in his
possession, books in French, Latin, Greek, Italian and
Spanish, that were bought at the sale of his effects, after
his death. He delighted chiefly in large books that
contained plates of any sort; and Gerard's large *Herbal*,
with wooden cuts, might be said to be his constant *vade
mecum*, which was displayed with much parade on the
table, or on the shelf, among other books of a like portly
appearance, to all his visitors ...

As the parish church was allowed to fall to ruin, and the
walls of the churchyard were kept up he made a practice
of frequenting that sequestered spot, by himself, where it
was not doubted but he held frequent converse with

departed spirits, who informed him of things that no mortal knowledge could teach ...

But it was not as a necromancer only that Adam Donald was consulted. He also acted as a physician. He was chiefly consulted in cases of lingering disorders, that were supposed to owe their origin to witchcraft, or some supernatural agency of this sort ... In these cases, he invariably prescribed the application of certain simple unguents of his own manufacture, to particular parts of the body, accompanied with particular ceremonies, which he described with all the minuteness he could; employing the most learned terms he could pick up to denote the most common things; so that, not being understood, the persons who consulted him, invariably concluded, when the cure did not succeed, that they had failed in some essential particular; and when the cure was effected he obtained full credit. Thus did his fame spread to the distance of thirty miles around him, in every direction; so that for a great many years of his life there was never a Sunday that his house was not crowded with visitors of various sorts, who came to consult him either as a necromancer, or physician. His fees were very moderate, never exceeding sixpence, when no medicines were given; and I believe a shilling was the very highest he ever obtained.[40]

It would be fascinating to know more about the actual 'unguents' that Adam used; but clearly his biographer was not particularly interested in them. The illustrations in Gerard's *Herbal* are stylized, and presumably Adam would have used the nearest approximation that he could find growing locally. It seems probable that his wandering around the churchyard, interpreted by his biographer as evidence of 'communing' with the dead, may in fact have been for the purposes of herb-gathering. Even today,

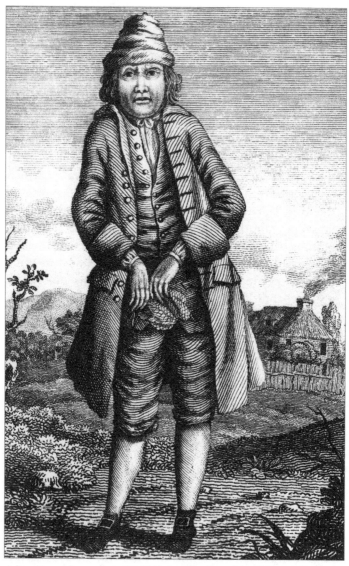

Adam Donald, prophet of Bethelnie, Aberdeenshire (1703–80). (From *The Bee*, vol. 6, 1791; NLS Shelfmark NH.295. Reproduced by permission of the Trustees of the National Library of Scotland)

churchyards are a rich source of varied local plants; in those days they would probably have been richer still. It seems likely that Adam relied heavily on the illustrations in Gerard's *Herbal*, since we know he could neither read nor write.

Indeed, one can speculate that the great success of Gerard's *Herbal*, and the prolonged period of time over which it has influenced practitioners of herbal medicine, could be due at least in part to its fine illustrations, from which the relatively poorly educated could recognize, in some cases, the familiar plants of their fields and hedgerows. Adam Donald is an example of someone who actually made a living from home-made herbal remedies; this is in contrast to the 'midwife-practitioner' whose services seem to have been free. Probably in some cases there was a system of barter, gifts of food, etc. being made in return for help given.

Janet Bell, who described herself as an apothecary, lived at Elsrickle, in Lanarkshire. Her family described her as 'airy-fairy', but even though she died as recently as 1880, it is very difficult to find out anything about her practice. In the photograph on p. 181 it looks as though there are several plants, presumably of the type she used in her practice. Probably there are no records of her practice because no records were ever made.

Sometimes there was only a fine dividing line between the local wise woman, or man, and the charlatans who exploited people's suffering and grew rich in the process. An example of a truly entrepreneurial spirit comes from North Walsham, Norfolk, in the late nineteenth century. Mrs Eliza Wesby was a 'doctress' at North Walsham between 1830 and 1865.[41] She produced a pamphlet in 1855 entitled *A Few Words of Friendly Advice*. The pamphlet consists largely of religious exhortations. On the first page she tells us that she has passed twenty-five years in the town and:

For many miles around there are people soliciting advice of me, although uneducated; and by doctoring wounds, and speaking on different events, I endeavour to support myself and my family. Many that know me, know that my lot is hard, for although my husband is an honest labouring man, it is seldom he has any employment.

Elsewhere in the same pamphlet she tells us:

I feel myself grateful to God for the mercies he has bestowed on me and on many that have called on me for advice. Through means of my medicine and the mercy of God, a great number who have lingered in ill health for many years are now enjoying good health; there are some who were thought incurable that are now quite restored ...

I prepare ointments of different kinds for green wounds, constitution sores, oils for the rheumatic sprains and weaknesses of the limbs. Corns cut and cures effected. Pills and cordials prepared from different herbs to suit the constitution in the spring and at leaf fall ...

I beg to inform the public at large that I shall continue my profession of doctress for the cure of all sorts of precarious diseases, such as the jaundice, weasing on the chest, trembling of the heart and many other nervous disorders that attend the human frame; also ulcers, sores and all manner of wounds. Ointments prepared, also an excellent linament for the Rheumatic.

I return my most humble thanks for the patronage I have received for the last twenty-five years I have been in practice.

Mrs Wesby's fame evidently lived on locally. The following anecdote about Mrs Wesby was recorded by Dr Mark Taylor, who was a Regional Health Officer in Norwich in the 1920s.

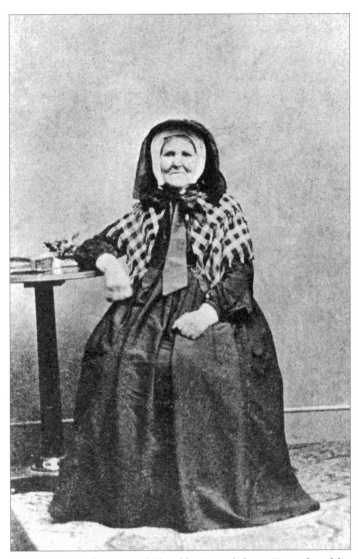

Janet Bell, 'apothecary', of Elsrickle, Lanarkshire. (Reproduced by permission of the Biggar Museum Trust)

Old Mrs Wesby of North Walsham used to give pills composed of paper on which texts of scripture were written. On being remonstrated with by the Vicar (previous to Canon Owen I think) she defended her practice by saying that 'it was in the Bible' and on being pressed to give locality, quoted '"the word of God is good for all things for doctrine and for instruction in righteousness", you give it for instruction in righteousness and I give it for doct'rin.'[42]

Fair enough!

Obviously the further we go back in time the more difficult it is to establish a true picture of the practitioners of herbal medicine. Undoubtedly there were quacks and charlatans in this field as in any other. Joanne Stevens made her fame and fortune during the eighteenth century by selling to Parliament her remedy for 'The Stone'.[43] Her cover could have been blown by a contemporary of hers, Sir John Clerk of Penicuik. In a mid-eighteenth-century manuscript written by him we read: 'but after all that was paid, I found the receipt in a little German Doctor's book printed in England in the Reign of Henry the 8th'.[44] When judging such stories, it should be borne in mind that many so-called 'charlatans' may have done just as much good as the orthodox physicians of the day. Since faith in a remedy always plays some part in its efficacy, it is rarely possible to dismiss any tried and tested remedy out of hand.

For some patients, a free remedy made from the infusion of a common wayside plant may be pre-judged as less effective than one bought from a chemist shop, or prescribed by a doctor. For others, the reverse may be true. The variety of medical treatments throughout the past three hundred years must at least to some extent reflect this variety in patient attitudes.

Undoubtedly there were a great many people with practical knowledge of the uses of everyday plants, and many of them put their knowledge to good use among their neighbours. Since, as we have seen, accurate written records of their remedies rarely survive, it is almost impossible to judge the efficacy of the remedies, let alone the motivation of the practitioners. Roy Palmer tells us: 'It has been suggested that 85% of those persecuted in the past as witches were wise women whose work was entirely beneficial, at least in intention.'[45] Our knowledge of this area is fragmentary at best, but of course even the everyday use of plant remedies could be abused. This is clearly illustrated in Chapter 1 by the case of Isobel F. from the records of the presbytery of Peebles. Although the case against her was considered unproven, she was accused of poisoning her husband by doctoring his ale with 'Badmonnie.'[46] Badmonnie is *Meum athamanticum*, of which Pechey wrote in 1694: 'It expels wind and forces Urine and the Courses ... Those that have vowed Chastity must not use it, for it is a great provocative to Venery.'[47] This plant grows in the mountains of Scotland and Wales, and was used in the Highlands as a vegetable.[48] Perhaps the Kirk Session felt that it was too harmless a plant to have been used as a murder weapon? The root smells aromatic and was apparently used as snuff.[49]

But on the whole, the use of native British plants as medicine formed part of inherited country lore for most families in the eighteenth century. Although there is rarely any written record of it, fragmentary information can sometimes be found, as in this description of an eighteenth-century Aberdeenshire hamlet:

About the place we find here and there an exceedingly rustic sort of garden. In these 'yards', which occur in no regular order ... may be found, besides certain useful vegetables, as 'kail', green or red, and 'syboes', a few old fashioned herbs and flowers. Some clusters of rich-scented honeysuckle, a plant of hardy southernwood, peppermint, and wormwood; with, mayhap, also a slip or two of 'smeird docken,' the sovereign virtues of whose smooth green leaves, in respect of sore fingers or broken shins, commend it to careful consideration.[50]

Was this the kind of garden to which Adam Donald had access? What are the plants mentioned here, and what were they used for? Even these simple questions cannot be answered with certainty.

Was the honeysuckle purely ornamental, or was it used, as in twentieth-century Hampshire,[51] to prepare an infusion for treating asthma? What were the 'syboes'? Again, was the southernwood (*Artemisia abrotanum*) mentioned actually used medicinally, or used as it was in this century in courtship,[52] or was it ornamental? Wormwood (*Artemisia absinthium*) was used in Scotland as a digestive aid, and a nerve tonic.[53] What is the identity of 'smeird docken'? The Scots Herbal gives 'smear docken' as a name for good King Henry (*Chenopodium bonus-henricus*): This plant was used as a pot herb in England and in Scotland: but was it used for sore shins and broken bones, or is this a case of mistaken identity? Was it in fact that common dock, whose leaves were used still in much more recent times for cuts and bruises?[54] This example serves to illustrate how, even when there is some kind of written record available on the subject of domestic plant medicine, it can sometimes leave numerous questions unanswered.

As we come forward in time, one might expect it to be easier to find out in more detail about the practitioners of herbal medicines, but this is not necessarily the case, again because few of them left any written record. Even our knowledge of twentieth-century plant medicine practitioners is extremely fragmentary. There are numerous tantalizing glimpses, as of Dido, a man of Romany extraction, living in Hainault Forest in the early years of the twentieth century:

> He was a very adroit man at making herbal medicine and ointments which cured whooping cough, measles, backache, liver trouble, burns etc ... From a fern, Dido made a green ointment which was very highly spoken of. This ointment apparently cured the chilblains of the Lambourne to Woodford bus driver. 'Dido said that the fern was getting very scarce – the only place left where he could find it was Loughton.'[55]

What was the identity of this fern? We may never know. I have questioned a Romany friend about the plant remedies used by his grandmother, and among them was an ointment for sore feet made from a fern, but again the identity of the fern is now unknown.

Frequently a fragment of information is preserved as a result of an individual's personal experience of the success of one particular plant remedy. For example, I was told of an impressively successful remedy for childhood eczema. The informant, now in his seventies, related how his brother had suffered miserably as a small child from eczema, which had made his life and his family's a misery. His mother was told to visit an old lady in Wivenhoe, who prepared a green ointment. The treatment was very successful, and when the ointment was finished, the mother returned to the old lady asking for more; instead, the lady told her how to make it; thereafter, whenever the child's eczema flared up, the ointment was used. This made such an impression on Mr H., that years later, when the daughter of a friend was suffering with eczema on her

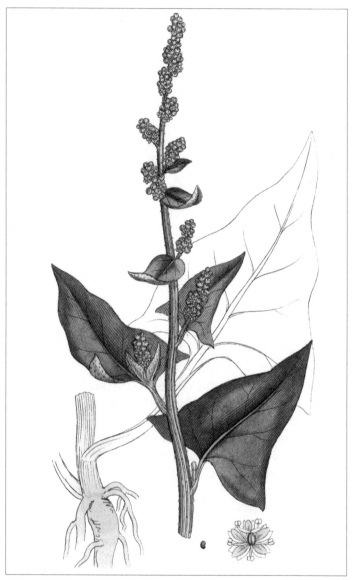

Good King Henry (*Chenopodium bonus-henricus*), from Sowerby's *English Botany*. (Photograph courtesy of John Innes Foundation Historical Collections)

hands, a condition that threatened her livelihood as a hairdresser, he told her about the remedy, and 'now I have a friend for life'![56]

Similarly, a striking plant remedy for dermatitis used with great success in the 1930s is the sole remedy remembered by an informant now living in Loddon, Norfolk. It was made from the root of a dock (*Rumex* sp.), and the informant had been given it by a man locally famous for his plant cures. Apparently, even the name of this local expert has been forgotten, and we shall probably never know what other remedies he used and suggested to others. It is sobering to reflect that, if so much twentieth-century knowledge of plant remedies has evidently been irretrievably lost, how much more must have been lost from previous centuries.

These examples of the type of person who used plant medicines in domestic medicine illustrate how in many parts of Britain, as recently as the early years of the twentieth century, plant medicines were a natural standby for many people in times of illness. Of course, there is an overlap between the plant medicines used in domestic medicine and those used by 'official' herbalists, but the two pharmacopoeias are not identical. One obvious difference is that in rural home medicine, locally available plants were used; in general this meant wild plants, and therefore native British plant species. Official medicine, whether we are considering orthodox medicine or herbalism, drew on a wider variety of plant species; indeed, one could argue that the more exotic a plant, the more worthwhile it might seem to be to the practitioners of orthodox medicine and to their relatively wealthy patients.

In the *Gunton Household Book*, written by several female generations of the Harbord family in Suffolk, there are several examples of complex remedies with innumerable costly ingredients. There are also examples of much simpler remedies and in some cases they are included as being suitable for 'the poor'. For example, the following is cited as suitable 'For a poor Country woman in Labour to hasten their birth':

> Take 3 handfulls of Mugwort, 12 cloves whole boyle them in a pint of white wine half an hour, then strein it and let the party drink it blood warm at a draught, you may gather Mugwort and dry it in a chamber and soe keep it all the year which is as usefull as the green is.[57]

The Harbord family were patients of Sir Thomas Browne, the famous Norfolk physician. A member of the Harbord family in labour would be likely to be treated with a much more complex array of ingredients. The heads of many country houses kept kitchen books in which they recorded culinary, household and medicinal recipes side by side. These often also include advice from friends, and information gathered from printed sources, such as magazines, newspapers and printed books. Even among the well-off, printed books were expensive, and evidently they were sometimes borrowed and copied.

Among the Clerk of Penicuik papers, there is a handwritten copy, 'Ane double', of the Receits of John Moncrief of Tippermalloch. In other instances, it is evident that material is copied from another source, but it has not proved possible to trace the source. A late seventeenth/early eighteenth-century manuscript that came to light in a Norfolk attic[58] has been beautifully transcribed from some other, presumably printed, source. A more recent example is a manuscript, written in the nineteenth century and now owned by a family in Colchester. On inspection, this appears to be a careful copy of some printed text on herbal remedies.

It is interesting to speculate that perhaps the line that divided an 'expert' from an ordinary user of plant remedies may have been the access to the printed word. Many of us had, and still have, possibly great respect for the printed word, so that an individual who combined the well-known traditional plant remedies with others obtained from books might have been regarded as more of an authority. I have frequently been struck by the fact that present-day informants on the subject of plant remedies often assume that only book knowledge is the kind required by me, rather than the traditional remedies handed down by word of mouth. Yet when one begins to analyse the sources of information contained in printed books, ironically it appears that many of them originally came from oral tradition; copied, and recopied, translated and sometimes modified and mis-stated, it becomes evident that the written record of plant medicine may sometimes be less accurate than the spoken.

5

MAGIC AND MEDICINE

If one were to believe the picture painted by Victorian folklorists, or by many orthodox medical practitioners, folk medicine consists of a quaint and entertaining collection of superstitious and ineffective remedies devised and used by those too ignorant to know better. Indeed, this description does fit quite closely the kind of folk medicine recorded in the literature. However, as we have seen in earlier chapters, the folk medicine as practised by the ordinary person in rural Britain was very largely devoid of ritual, superstition and magic, and usually involved the use of one or a few readily available common British plants. So why has folk medicine become so misrepresented?

The reasons are various. One is the gulf between the users and the recorders of domestic remedies. Not only was an element of patronization present at least until and sometimes well into the twentieth century: in addition, there was often a total lack of understanding. Domestic medicine is one aspect of the ordinary daily life of country people. There was, and is, no motivation for the users of domestic medicine to record their remedies in print. What little writing there is on the subject has usually been written by people with no direct experience of country remedies. This not only removes the information from its context, it also tends to lead to condescending attitudes towards the users of such remedies.

The very word 'folk' has come to have a patronizing ring to it, and too often accounts of folk medicine concentrate on the bizarre and the fanciful. Remedies taken out of context, and sometimes even misquoted, have built up a picture of folk medicine as a collection of odd anachronistic rituals, practised by the ignorant and superstitious. In reality, domestic medicine was a necessary tool for survival, and still is in many countries. It is a home survival kit, built up over many centuries and orally preserved from one generation to the next. It represents the distilled plant wisdom of many centuries, and it is our loss if we dismiss this wisdom too lightly.

As Thompson has pointed out, history written by the labouring classes would read very differently from that written by the cultural elite. Too much history, he says, is 'a description of social relations as they may be seen from above'.[1] A few folklorists have always been aware of this. Gomme pointed out that 'great masses of people do not belong to the civilization which towers over them and which is never of their creation'.[2] Likewise, a history of domestic medicine written by its users would undoubtedly read very differently from the Victorian accounts of 'Folk Medicine'. Domestic medicine was largely the province of women, and even less is known about their daily life in the past than about the life of men.[3] It is hardly surprising that no reliable written record of domestic plant medicine exists in this century; in Thompson's words, 'the labouring poor did not leave their workhouses stashed with documents for historians to work over'.[4] Ewart Evans described the oral tradition in East Anglia as 'the voice of a class of people that have had little opportunity to speak for themselves'.[5]

The only records we have of this empirical first aid are glimpses, recorded incidentally in such works as the herbals and later the Floras of Britain. Otherwise we have to depend on the more biased writers of folklore, and the recording of some weird or ritualistic method of healing makes for more exciting reading than that of a down-to-earth plant remedy. Nor are the authors of these works necessarily responsible for inaccurate reporting. It is an occupational hazard for the oral historian that one will be told what one wants (or expects) to hear. While speaking to one of Ewart Evans' informants on the subject of the famous (or infamous) use of toad bones in taming a horse,[6] I was told, 'We told him what he wanted to hear.' I asked if this was what they were doing with me, and was assured to the contrary; but who knows? All too often we are probably misled in this way. Indeed, it has often struck me as very surprising that people have been as forthcoming as they often have with me. Why should some elderly person brought up in conditions of hardship that I could hardly visualize be willing to talk to me, with my middle-class background and educated accent so clearly showing! The oral historian seeks to drop into a stranger's life and expects to share their recollections. It has been a repeated pleasant surprise to find how readily many people have shared their knowledge. However, I am aware that no one is immune to having the wool pulled over his or her eyes!

Deliberate deception apart, there are other factors, such as the repetition of printed errors, which make our record of domestic medicine inaccurate as well as incomplete. An undue respect for the printed word, enhanced by the scarcity and expense of books in the past, has encouraged ordinary people to devalue their own knowledge of plant medicine.

In earlier chapters there are numerous examples of instructions that were intended to define the time of harvesting or the place to gather the plant; both these factors can have an important effect on the efficacy of the remedy. The gathering of plants from shady places, or in the springtime, is not part of some weird ritual; it is evidence of the accurate observation by our ancestors of the variability in effectiveness of plants throughout the season and in different environments. For example, in the following recipe for nettle broth recorded from the Highlands by Marian McNeil,[7] a sensible place from which to gather the nettles is specified: 'Gather young nettles from the higher part of the wall where they are clean. Wash the tops in salted water and chop very finely ...' Nettles have been eaten in this way for many centuries; they even appear in songs and proverbs, such as the famous Renfrewshire saying[8] quoted on p. 125, stressing its value as a tonic. And Chambers, in his *Popular Rhymes of Scotland*, quotes the following poem:

> Gin ye be for lang kail
> Cou' the nettle, stoo the nettle
> Gin ye be for lang kail,
> Cou' the nettle early[9]

The instructions embodied in these quotations mean that only the young shoots of the nettle plants will be used, and these only in the first half of the year. It is known now that the older parts of the nettle plant are toxic, and that it is inadvisable to eat nettles later in the year when all parts of the plant can be toxic. This was evidently known empirically long before it was confirmed by modern science.

Many such examples quoted in the literature of the association of ritual and magic with plant healing prove on closer inspection to be remnants of practical instructions that have been largely ratified by modern science. So why have 'Old Wives' Tales' come to have such a bad reputation, as being fanciful, full of magic ritual and superstition? Most people judge these remedies by what they have read about them. But the recorders of these remedies were not the users of them, and those who recorded them, whether in ancient manuscripts such as *Herbarium Apuleii* or in nineteenth century folklore books, were catering for a literate audience, which immediately excludes a large proportion of the users of domestic remedies. A dry list of plant remedies would have little appeal as a work of literature. These authors were appealing to the side of human nature that likes magic and mystery and religion, and therefore emphasized the strange, mysterious and bizarre, which make for more exciting reading than the plain remedies.

Moreover, the authors of works on popular or traditional medicine rarely distinguish between the self-help remedies and those used by healers. Accompanying charms and incantations filled a different role to the simple plant remedies, and were probably used, in so far as they were used at all, by individuals who presented themselves as healers, not as part of self-treatment. Recourse to a healer was a step taken after home remedies had failed; if the practical everyday solution was inadequate, then it might prove worthwhile consulting a higher authority. This healer must be seen to have knowledge over and above the common knowledge of plant remedies. The healer must dispense that extra ingredient along with the medicine: prayer in the case of the monk or the clergyman, magic or charms in the case of the conjuror or white witch. To inspire faith in the patient, the healer must be seen as possessing special knowledge or special power or both. This is the beginning of the patient-healer relationship, and it is worth stressing that its formation is a mutual process, elicited by the sufferer and accepted or actively encouraged by the healer.

Once a healer is involved, the role of ritual and magic becomes more important. Self-help medicine is in general free from such ritual. An analogy would be that a person eating a meal on his own may well eat off a plate on his lap. Eating in a restaurant in company, the meal is far more of a ritual, with tablecloths, candles and flowers, not simply a plateful of food. The link that is so often made in the literature between traditional medicine and magic applies mainly to cases where a healer is involved. In the literature, self-medication has been largely ignored, yet it was probably the first response of most country people in Britain in times of accident or illness.[10] Such self-reliance was born out of necessity, and has survived as a quality of many country people through to the present era. Here are some examples taken from twentieth-century East Anglians:

Old Jan was quite a character! A small, wizened woman, her features bronzed with many years exposure to all types of weather. Her movements, despite her years, were quick with an agility more common to someone half her age, which was widely rumoured to be in the region of seventy-five years ...

Several years have gone since Jan passed over, but five years before her death I had the good fortune to be in her company, and to be entrusted with some of her 'old fashioned remedies'. It happened that she was potato-picking for us, and about the middle of the morning it started raining, stopping potato-lifting. We all adjourned into the barn, and the conversation turned to the newly instituted National Health Service. Jan insisted, 'We don't need all these 'ere doctors, we can look after ourselfs.' She then straightway launched into a list of complaints and their treatment, some of which I hereby reveal below:

Cuts, abrasions and fleshwounds

After stemming the flow of blood, apply a dried dock leaf liberally treated with brandy, and bandage tightly. Change the dressing each day until the wound heals

Housemaids Knee

Prepare a poultice. Take half a pound of ground linseed, cover with boiling water. Strain off the water, and place linseed in a calico bag. Apply the bag to the knee as hot as the patient can bear it, and bandage. All swelling and pain should be gone within seven days.[11]

Other remedies used by Jan included such household remedies as oil of cloves for toothache, eucalyptus oil for sore throat, and a poultice of breadcrumbs, sugar and egg white for 'festering' wounds. Although such household remedies are not strictly plant medicines, they are of interest as examples of practical self-treatment and illustrate the type of self-reliance possessed by many country people, a quality dramatically illustrated by the story of a Norfolk woman who poulticed both her broken wrists with comfrey, rather than going to hospital (p. 43). To many country people, hospital was a last resort, rather than a first recourse. A story is also told of a Suffolk man advised to attend hospital who complained that he didn't feel well enough![12] It was probably the quality of self-reliance characteristic of many country people in the past which, combined with necessity, initially led to the discovery of numerous cheap and easily accessible domestic plant remedies, which became part of common knowledge, handed down from one generation to the next. In common with other traditions, they were both taken for granted and respected. Along with which plants to use for which ailment, and how to prepare a given remedy, information was probably also passed down concerning the effectiveness or otherwise of a particular remedy. While they were the only form of treatment available, such plant remedies would have been used, as being better than nothing, regardless of their efficacy.

Further examples are provided by Rolf, the self-styled King of the Norfolk Poachers, who wrote down some of his life's memories when he was seventy-five years old, to be published as a book in 1935. As a child, he spent a lot of time with his grandparents, whose company he obviously preferred to that of his religious and strait-laced father:

> My old Granny was a bit of a quack Doctor, and the People used to come to her with all there ills. She was a mid Wife beside, and one to help with the layen out of Boddies. She told me all the Charms and such like that I know, and lernt me lots of old songs and sayens that was goen about in them days, I suppose that some of them was two hundred years old. I can rember some of them but I have never seen them riten down ...
>
> My grandmother had a cure of sorts for evrything, and herbs for evry complaint.[13]

This phrase 'herbs for evry complaint' sums up the role of plant remedies in rural life in the past, and it is significant that Rolf distinguishes between these (common-sense) remedies and the charms used for a wide variety of ailments. He continues:

> The olden time People used a lot of Charms for rhumatics, and they do still in many parts. One would carry the bone of the Pig's foot in there pockets, it was the Bone that

Joined the foot to the ankle of the pig. Another would carry the first new Potato, the size of a small egg in his, and another a pice of stone sulphur. A very favrite cure was a pice of brass, a pice of Zinc and a pice of Copper in a bag, wich must be worn on the sufferer. Some would put new flanel next the skin and wear it till it would hold on no more.

Evidently Rolf's Granny used plant remedies like everybody else, but in addition she built up a reputation for herself as a healer and used charms as well. Such healers are the ones who are portrayed in folklore literature as the typical user of herbs. This is far from being the case. The typical user of herbs was the ordinary country person who could not afford medical help for his daily ailments and used the plants around him in the same way that his family had for generations. If his own methods of self-help failed, then he would consult a local expert, such as Rolf's Granny.

Most written records concern the practice of healers, practice that incorporated herbal knowledge but added to it elements of magic, mystery, secrecy, religion or all four. Such healers sometimes made a good living out of their practice. The famous sixteenth-century herbalist and surgeon Gerard distinguishes in his *Herball* between the different users of plant remedies. After describing a remedy for treating wounds, he tells the reader:

I send this jewell unto you women of all sorts, especially those such as cure and helpe the poore and impotent of your countrey without reward. But unto the beggarly rabble of witches, charmers, and such like couseners, that regard more to get money, than to helpe for charitie, I wish these few medicines far from their understanding, and from those deceivers, whom I wish to be ignorant herein.[14]

The use of plants as self-help remains now largely a fading memory in the minds of elderly country people: it is an oral tradition that is rapidly coming to an end. This is another reason why the picture of domestic plant medicine in Britain has become falsified. Time and again, I have been told of an elderly relative who knew the uses of plants for healing, but the present-day informant has forgotten which plant was used for what; through disuse, many of the ordinary remedies have fallen into oblivion.

A lady mentioned in Chapter 4 (p. 165) inherited a cottage from a much-loved aunt. The cottage is situated on an area of marshy common-land, very rich in plant diversity. The present owner told me that though her aunt knew the uses of every plant growing on the common, she herself remembers only a handful of plant remedies.[15] There must be countless stories like this.

How far have we misinterpreted the role of the 'wise man', 'cunning man' or 'wise woman' of the past? Perhaps many of them were the equivalent of this informant's aunt: well-versed in plant medicines, and therefore able to help family and friends in time of sickness; just this and no more: there may have been no ritual or magic in their home medicines. This is not to deny the existence of magical and ritualistic practices in medicine. To deny this would be to fly in the face of the evidence. What I am suggesting is that family plant medicine was relatively free of these elements. Indeed, the use of native plants in self-help medicine in this country may have been the one constant thread in the history of medical practice. Magical and religious and astrological practices associated with physic waxed and waned in popularity, but the use of 'simples' remained constant: a standby for country people in times of illness.

Those wealthy enough to have a choice could draw on traditional knowledge or have recourse to a healer. Even so, as late as the eighteenth century even members of the gentry might choose self-help, as, for example, when Christian Kilpatrick, wife of Sir John Clerk of Penicuik, wrote to him that she intended giving her son a saffron and marigold posset to treat his smallpox (p. 71).[16]

Orthodox medical treatment at the time included blood-letting, purging, blistering plasters, as well as a range of polypharmaceutical medicines. Home treatment may have been preferable for the patient, a view echoed in the ballad of Lord Livingstone:

> O live, O live, Lord Livingston
> The space o ae half hour
> There's nae a leech in Edinbro town
> But I'll bring to your door
>
> Awa wi your leeches, lady, he said
> Of them I'll be the waur
> There's nae a leech in Edinbro town
> That can strong death debar[17]

In other instances, simple home remedies were tried by the wealthy when official medicine had failed. The following eighteenth-century letter illustrates this:

As my dear boy is the most interesting subject to me, I shall begin with him ... When the medicine of Dr Cullen failed, I shall give him garlic in brandy ... I shall engage it will free him of worms. and it is attended with no inconvenience, but his breath will perfume the air.[18]

It is interesting to note that Mrs S.W. informs me that the same remedy was still in use in rural Suffolk, 220 years later.[19]

In the diary of George Ridpath, a mid-eighteenth-century minister in Stitchel, we read:

Munday May 2nd 1757
sore distrest at a pain and stiffness in the lowere ribs ...

Thursday May 5th ... easier today, tho' still greatly opprest. Drank in the morning ground ivy with dandelion and betony, and a little lavender to flavour them. Finding these things clearing my crop gradually, and promoting a diuresis.[20]

Faced with a wide variety of incurable diseases, the healer, whether an orthodox practitioner or a quack, had to offer some new element of treatment other than the well-known plant remedies. Presumably this was the reason for the development within official medicine of more and more complex combinations of plant medicines, as well as for the importation of exotic and expensive plant and animal ingredients. Gerard (1545–1607) comments on this liking for the new and exotic. After discussing the herb goldenrod (*Solidago virgaurea*), used for staunching bleeding, he relates:

In my remembrance I have known the dry herbe which came from beyond the sea sold in Bucklersbury for halfe a crowne an ounce. But since it was found in Hampstead wood, even as it were at our townes end, no man will give halfe a crowne for an hundred weight of it: which plainely setteth forth our inconstancie and sudden mutabilitie, esteeming no longer of anything, how pretious soever it be, than whilest it is strange and rare. This verifieth our English proverbe, Far fetcht and deare bought is best for Ladies. Yet it may be more truely said of phantasticall Physitions, who when they have found an approved medicine and perfect remedy neere home against any

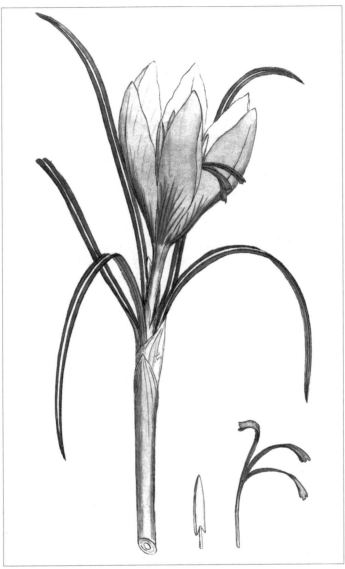

Saffron (*Crocus sativus*), from Sowerby's *English Botany*. (Photograph courtesy of John Innes Foundation Historical Collections)

disease: yet not content therewith, they will seeke for a new further off, and by that meanes many times hurt more than they helpe. Thus much I have spoken to bring these new fangled fellowes backe again to esteeme better of this admirable plant than they have done, which no doubt have the same virtue now that then it had, although it growes so neere our owne homes in never so great quantity.[21]

For some patients in the past, as at the present time, traditional plant remedies were held in great esteem and gave them independence in times of illness. Others had overmuch respect for the novel or exotic remedy: this was the group of patients who brought about the development of official polypharmacy. Official medicine could only develop along those lines dictated by the paying patient.

The eighteenth-century Scottish surgeon-apothecary, mentioned in Chapter 1, who prescribed nettles for his patient, 'knowing how she dislik'd all shop med'cines'[22] was recognizing this fact. There are, and probably always have been, a variety of attitudes among people of all social classes towards the use of self-medication and towards the traditional plant medicines employed by country people in the past. The Dalkeith patient mentioned above probably represents the eighteenth-century equivalent of Nan whose fierce self-dependence and respect for the old traditional ways is illustrated on p. 131. Others react against the old familiar ways and have added respect for anything that is new, or expensive. These are the people at whom advertising of all sorts is successfully aimed.

Because new and exotic remedies are more costly than the traditional home remedies, they will be mainly used by the better-off members of society, for whom a greater choice in medical treatment is available. One would expect the kitchen books of the wealthy to reflect this

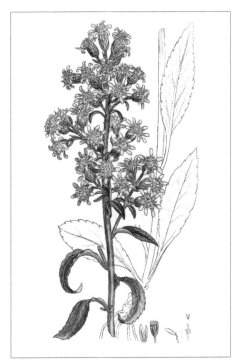

Golden rod (*Solidago virgaurea*), from Sowerby's *English Botany*. (Photograph courtesy of John Innes Foundation Historical Collections)

greater choice, and this is indeed the case. During the eighteenth century in Britain when the majority of rural workers could not afford medical aid, their remedies seem to have consisted mainly of simple plant remedies, or indeed of non-plant household remedies. The rural East Anglian, as recently as the early decades of the twentieth century, used urine to treat chilblains. The Harbord family, wealthy landowners in Norfolk, used wine for the same complaint!

The kitchen books kept by successive generations of the Harbord family make fascinating reading, and the practical details supplied with some recipes suggest those that were actually used. One example is quoted on p. 35. Here is another instance where the detail suggests a remedy that was actually prepared and used rather than only recorded:

> Broom flowers and elder flowers in fresh butter, stood in the sun, make an ointment for a Wen being well rubbed in with a warm hand, for a strain or a burn for shrinking of a Vein or Sinews or any swellings, for splints in a horse or swelling in a cow's teat.[23]

As would be expected, those remedies showing evidence of actual use tend to be simpler, and cheaper, than those copied from official contemporary medicine. Compare these two remedies for whooping cough:

> Figg drink is one of ye best things for a hoping cough to strike into childrens mouths with a feather as they sleep.

> *Sir Tho: Browns drink for a hoping Cough*
> Take of Raysons of ye Sunn ston'd an Ounce Currance a Spoonfull, 5 or 6 figgs, 8 or 9 Coltsfoot leaves marrygold and Cowslip flowers of each a few, Liquorich a quarter of an ounce, Aniseeds a thimble full, China roots a quarter of an ounce, boyle all these in a pint and a half of Barly water to a pint, then strein it and give it 2 or 3 spoonfulls at a time warme when you see reason, adding to it a little syrup of Violets or Sugar Candy its good without either.[24]

It seems likely that the simple fig drink would have been the remedy actually used in practice. Contrast the ingredients of these two remedies: 'For the Stone and Cholick aproved, Inward bark of ash boiled in white wine.' Meanwhile, 'Sir Tho Brown's drink for the Stone in ye kidneys and bloody Urine' includes Marshmallow roots, Eringo roots, Asparagus, Liquorish, Red Sanders, French barley, Fennel seed, Quince seed, honey, water and yeast.[25]

Self-medication, whether among rich or poor, was likely to employ simpler remedies than those prescribed by a healer of any kind.

Through such kitchen books it is sometimes possible to obtain glimpses of the 'folk' medicine practised by country people. A nineteenth-century Norfolk manuscript includes the following two recipes:

For a Consumption
Two handfuls of Water Cresses boiled in a quart of spring water till it comes to a pint
1 teacupful every morning before he gets out of bed: he will be cured in nine mornings
This was given by a Gypsey to a Person in a Consumption, and effected a Cure

For Dropsy
6 oz Horse Radish cut in slices, 4 oz of the best Ginger sliced Two Handfuls of stinging nettles, to be boiled in two quarts of Water till it comes to one, then to be strained off, and a bottle of the best Gin put into it, and just simmer'd up to be well mixed, then to be put away and bottled. One wineglassfull to be taken an hour before Breakfast, another two hours before Dinner.

This Receipt was given me by an old Woman who assured me she had cured several Persons who had been attended by Medical Men without receiving any benefit.[26]

The notes in an eighteenth-century Flora relate that one of the Newmarket huntsman of James II told the king of a cure for the bite of a mad dog, which uses 'star of the earth'[27] (probably *Plantago coronopus*, although there seems to have been some confusion over its identity[28]). There is the following note written by Sir James Cullum in his own copy of Hudson's *Flora Anglica*, regarding

'Leontodon Taraxacum' (i.e. dandelion): 'Old Gordon the Gardener informs me that he has himself experienced the chewing the dried roots a very great Relief in the Asthma 13 Sep 1777.'[29]

Apart from occasional overlaps, such as the *Gunton Household Book* remedy 'For a poor Country Woman in Labour' mentioned on p. 188,[30] it seems that the traditional use of plant remedies stayed as a separate, orally preserved tradition, upon which official contemporary medical practice had little effect. However, the early herbals date from a time when there was still considerable overlap between the actual plants used in home medicine and in orthodox medicine; and in these we find references to country remedies. But, as time progressed, the Materia Medica of official medicine diverged more and more from that of the ordinary country person, so that by the eighteenth century such manuals of self-help as William Buchan's *Domestic Medicine*[31] represent distilled orthodox medicine, far removed from the self-help practised by ordinary country people.

Although Wesley's *Primitive Physick* was an attempt to bring medical help to the masses, it was drawn largely from the writings of orthodox medical men such as Boerhaave, Sydenham, Cheyne and others. The author, in a postscript to the 1755 edition,[32] states his intention: 'to set down cheap and safe easy medicines, easily to be known, easy to be procured, and easy to be applied by plain unlettered men'. Yet even this book was obviously available to the illiterate only indirectly through their patrons and, while its remedies resemble traditional ones in being simpler than many orthodox medical prescriptions, the book draws largely on earlier printed sources.

Since traditional country remedies were and are preserved almost entirely by oral tradition it is almost impossible to establish the attitude of most of their users both to the official medicine of the day and to their own familiar remedies. If we take oral historical evidence into account, and view twentieth-century country remedies as the end of this long traditional line, then it seems that such remedies were not part of a 'system' of healing, nor were they the product of religious or magical theories of disease. Rather, they were a first-aid response to illness, an integral and unquestioned part of country life. If such simple remedies failed, then recourse might be had to a local healer, who according to circumstance and geography might be a local wise man or woman, a member of the clergy or of the gentry, or a member of the medical profession. It is when the healer intervenes that rituals of magic and religion enter into the picture. It is the confusion between self-treatment with country remedies and their use by a wide variety of healers that has led to the widespread image of plant medicine as associated with magic, both black and white, and with superstition.

The most famous, (or infamous) example of the image given to plant medicine is the doctrine of signatures, already mentioned in Chapter 1. This supposes that God has indicated in the features of a plant what its medical uses to mankind might be: thus lungwort (*Pulmonaria officinalis*) with the spotted leaves was good for diseased lungs, and the leaves of poplar (*Populus* spp.) quake in the wind so were good for shaking palsy. Among the most famous exponents of this doctrine is Paracelsus, whose actual name was Theophrastus von Bombastus (1493–1541). He was a doctor, and a professor at Basle, unpopular with his colleagues and evidently eccentric. As a Neoplatonist, Paracelsus was interested in the ideas of macrocosm and microcosm; his doctrine of signatures needs to be seen in this context, as part of the reflection of the divine plan in the organization of the world. In his own words: 'the physician should also study the lines of the herbs and the leaves, and by the application of chiromancy, he should discover their efficacy and virtues.'[33]

The idea was adopted by many others, notably Porta in Naples and later, in England, by William Coles and Nicholas Culpeper (1616–54). An example of the extremes to which this idea was taken is to be found in the writing of Richard Sanders, who described himself as a student in the Divine and Celestial Sciences. In the preface to the first edition of his book, *Physiognomie and Chiromancie*, he expounds the doctrine of signatures, although his analogies seem to struggle!

> Plants which resemble the figure of the heart have the power and vertue of comforting and sustaining the heart; as the Citron apple, the fruit of Anacardus, like the heart; Fuller's thistle, Spikenard, Balm, Mint, the White Beet, Trifoly, Parsly and Motherwort, which bear in leaves and roots the physiognomie of the heart, and are comfortive thereunto ... the leaves of Water Mint resembling the nose, yield an extract wonderful good for the recovery of that sense ... Herbs whose acidity turns milk into curd, profit much as to generation; such as the herb Gallium, or Cheese rennet, and the seeds of Spurge.[34]

The doctrine of signatures was adopted by many sixteenth- and seventeenth-century writers, including Robert Turner, who states that 'God hath imprinted upon the Plants, Herbs, and Flowers, as it were in Hieroglyphicks, the very signature of their Vertues'.[35]

What was the origin of the doctrine of signatures? Was Paracelsus actually re-interpreting a much earlier collection of mnemonics that helped illiterate users of plant remedies to remember which plant was useful for which ailment? This is a plausible possibility. Is the so-called doctrine of signatures a distortion by the learned, another instance where 'They books, they get it all wrong' (see p. 30). It would seem likely that a country person seeking a particular plant to treat his ailment would use any feature of the plant to remind himself which plant to use. Pilewort is not useful for treating piles *because* it has tuber-like projections; but this is a convenient way of remembering which plant to gather for treating piles. The common name of a plant in many cases serves to remind people of its use, too, as in the case of Pilewort.

Leon Petulengro, describing his own Romany boyhood in Norfolk, relates how his father explained to him that the plant *names* 'were similar to the disease. Chestnut leaves for the chest complaints; gravel root (*Eupatorium purpureum*) for stone and gravel; liverwort for the liver; lungwort for lungs; heart'sease for weak hearts, and even the herb called rupturewort (*Herniaria* sp.) will ease rupture. He taught me to recognize these.'[36] Clearly, plant names were used as reminders of their medicinal properties, and it seems plausible to suggest that physical features of the plant would have been used similarly.

The actual users of domestic plant remedies had neither spare time nor education; consideration of any doctrines, religious or otherwise, was and still is a luxury for the better off. The ideas of the learned probably have little impact on the daily lives of the rest of humanity. It seems likely that the so-called doctrine of signatures propounded by Paracelsus and adopted by many other medical practitioners in Britain would have had little impact on the mass of ordinary people. Indeed, even religious doctrine often fails to filter down to the ordinary people. Keith Thomas quotes the fourteenth-century preacher, John Bromyard, who used to relate the story of a shepherd who, asked if he knew who the Father, Son and Holy Ghost were, replied, 'The father and the son I know well for I tend their sheep, but I know not that third fellow: there is none of that name in our village.'[37]

What an irony then that the doctrine of signatures is often cited as an example of the ignorance and naivety of country people. Yet the doctrine was formulated not by a user of plant remedies in folk medicine but by a learned member of the medical profession.

Once Paracelsus' doctrine had been expounded, quoted and re-quoted in the literature, it became the stuff of quasi-folk medicine, and may even have fed back into the folk tradition. However, it does seem likely that originally it was an inversion of an empirical finding by country people, a distortion produced by the learned, and subsequently used to ridicule the traditions of the unlearned. The one benefit of the adoption of the doctrine of signatures by men of learning is that it has preserved the knowledge of some plant remedies which might otherwise have been lost. Unfortunately, it is also one of the factors that has produced an entirely false picture in the literature of what was a common-sense collection of plant medicines.

Another falsifying element in the record of domestic plant medicine has been the gradual decline in the use of country medicines. Once a practice has fallen from use, the details of it quickly become confused, and eventually distorted or lost all together. A twentieth-century example will serve to illustrate the way in which practical instructions for using plants could easily be misconstrued as superstition and ritual. A Norfolk man in the 1930s was suffering from dermatitis, which had been diagnosed and unsuccessfully treated at a local hospital. Neighbours told him to consult a man locally famous for his knowledge of plants. He was told to go to the marshes behind his house, and to dig up some dock roots, but *only to select those plants growing with their feet in the water* (my italics). He did as suggested, made an ointment from the dock roots, and used it to successfully treat his dermatitis. His family were so impressed that they regularly made up a batch of this ointment, and used it themselves and supplied it to friends. It was found to be effective in treating any skin rashes, including those resulting from childhood vaccinations.[38] It would be easy to dismiss the specific instruction regarding the location of the dock roots as superstitious ritual. However, the true marsh dock (*Rumex palustris*) is not a common plant, and the marshes in this area are one of the localities in which it has been recorded in the past.[39] So was the adviser suggesting that the actual water dock was used, rather than the common dock? Unfortunately this cannot be proved, since the marshland concerned has now been drained, but it could be the case.

Of course it would not be true to say that all use of plant medicines was or is devoid of magic and superstition; but these are probably later accretions to an originally empirical use. In a study of herbal remedies for livestock used in the seventeenth and eighteenth centuries, Drury found that although certain plants such as rowan (*Sorbus aucuparia*) and elder (*Sambucus nigra*) are associated with magical traditions, there is little by way of ritual accompanying internal herbal remedies.[40] There are innumerable examples of charms and rituals associated with plant healing from Anglo-Saxon times onwards, but these seem to have been associated with the practice of healers, rather than with self-medication. Susan Palliser regards the ritual surrounding plant medicine as having a twofold use; incorporating practical instruction and ratifying by a deity.[41] It does seem likely that this latter is an added accretion, whose importance will vary in time and space.

An effective home remedy probably does not require accompanying ritual, religious or otherwise. A tried and tested remedy would need no accompaniment. One could argue that those illnesses that fail to respond to simple home treatment would be the ones for which the sufferer had recourse to a healer, and to religion, and to anything else that might help. In the case of failure of home treatment, the courses open to the sufferer would depend on his or her social standing as well as location. For the poor country dweller, a local expert would probably be the next port of call: for the wealthy, official medical aid could be sought. To what extent magic, superstition and religion would enter in at this stage would depend on the individual's circumstances and inclination.

However, within the Celtic tradition, it is more likely that magico-religious elements of healing have played a greater part than in the rest of Britain, and the remnants of this can still be seen today: Mary Beith gives numerous examples of healing ritual from the Highlands of Scotland;[42] the famous physicians of Myddfai in Wales were families of healers who combined plant medicine with magic and superstition;[43] and in Ireland, it is still possible to find examples of ritualistic healers.[44] In England, it is difficult if not impossible to ascertain the extent to which 'witchcraft' and superstition was actually associated with healing; we have to rely on accounts written by biased authors, often by members of the medical profession. It seems probable that many women described as witches were innocent practitioners of herbal medicine: others undoubtedly cultivated the image of witchcraft so that they had more to offer their customers than the common knowledge of plant medicines.

Another important point is that the sixteenth- and seventeenth-century works that refer to the 'common people' and their beliefs are written by people who consider themselves superior in education. How often are the thoughts and beliefs of the common people totally misrepresented as a result? There is often an unwritten *assumption* that certain beliefs are held in common: often this does not bear close scrutiny. Thomas provides numerous examples of the falsity of this assumption, such as Pemble's story of the seventeenth-century man questioned about his religious beliefs:

> being demanded what he thought of God, he answers that he was a good old man; and what of Christ, that he was a towardly young youth; and of his soul, that it was a great bone in his body; and what should become of his soul after he was dead, that if he had done well he should be put into a pleasant green meadow.[45]

Writers on the subject assure us that the mass of people in rural Britain resorted to witches for healing, divination and sorcery. What the common people really thought about such matters can only be a matter of guesswork. It is significant that the seventeenth-century manuscript entitled *The Winnowing of White Witchcraft* is written by a contemporary member of the medical profession. It takes the form of a conversation between 'Dr Dreadnought, a Divine, Phylomathes, a physition and Gregory Grosshead, a country corydon' and contains phrases such as 'the common people do much reqyert white witches and are ready to make apologies for them' and 'the common people, are for the most part ignorant, and know not what prayer is'. Elsewhere the author refers to 'the sottish conceit of many country people who thinke that white witches are illumined from above'. White witches, we are told 'are without learning for the most part and use unlawful means'. The doctor accuses white witches of having 'few salves and medicines for manifold malladies'.

Repeated several times throughout the manuscript is the statement that 'the common sorte think it to be no sinn to goe unto white witches'.[46]

Now all this adds up to a clearly biased account. To what extent did the common people really resort to witches? To what extent were these so-called witches dabbling in the supernatural, and to what extent were they harmless dispensers of herbal medicines? We shall probably never know. Writing in 1584, Reginald Scott tells us 'it is indifferent to say in the English tongue, "she is a witch" or "she is a wise woman"'.[47]

This confusion presumably persisted. Thomas quotes the case of a woman near Cambridge accused, in 1592, of being a cunning woman. She defended herself, saying that 'she doth not use any charms, but that she doth use ointments and herbs to cure many diseases'.[48]

It is very difficult to guess whether the popular image of witchcraft today represents the continuation of a long-held belief, or whether it is a mish-mash of ideas, influenced as much by Grimm's *Fairy Tales* as by any real racial memory of the powers of witchcraft. Much is the stuff of children's fairy tales, and it is quite possible that many wise women branded as witches in the past were as harmless, and indeed helpful, as the two old ladies locally regarded as witches in the twentieth century (p. 164).

This book is about self-help using plants, and to attempt to survey the whole field of supernatural healing would be totally inappropriate, but it is interesting to consider to what extent faith, with a small or a capital 'F', entered into the use of plant medicines by ordinary country people. A recent example of this is provided by the childhood memories of a lady brought up in the Romney marshes, mentioned in Chapter 3, who recalls her mother's recipe for cabbage water as a cure for rheumatism 'with faith'.[49] Belief in the effectiveness of a remedy undoubtedly increases its healing effect: otherwise there would be no such thing as the well-known and well-documented placebo effect. This is true whether the remedy is a plant plucked from the hedgerow, a charm pronounced by a healer, or a prescription written by a modern orthodox practitioner. Presumably, the objectively more effective remedy will need less accompanying faith than the less effective one. Some illnesses seem to be more susceptible to 'faith-healing' than others; and some individuals are more suggestible than others. All these factors have, consciously or otherwise, been exploited by healers throughout the world.

It would be interesting to know whether illnesses regarded as incurable were more often taken to a healer in the past than those which responded readily to home medication. Presumably this would be the case; fragments of twentieth-century oral historical evidence suggest that, as the century progressed, domestic plant remedies for cancer, for example, became less frequent: but this could merely reflect the improvement in orthodox treatment available to all since the advent of the National Health Service.

6

WARTS AND ALL

Considering that warts are not normally a serious medical condition, it is at first sight difficult to understand why the subject of warts seems to have attracted so much interest. Wart remedies are numerous, very varied, and sometimes bizarre. The home treatment for most trivial ailments is often a very simple common-sense remedy, but for warts the picture is quite different; it seems that there is no limit to the credulity of mankind when dealing with wart cures.

Why should warts form a category on their own in this respect? Is it because they are somewhat mysterious, appearing and disappearing apparently without rhyme or reason? Is it because they represent a slight social stigma; they are often the subject of jokes, or even proverbs (as in 'warts and all', originating from Oliver Cromwell). Or is it simply because everyone likes a little mystery and magic, and warts are a fertile area for unexplained cures?

In an attempt to give an overall picture of the traditional treatments for warts, the remedies tried will be divided into those using plants, those using animals or animal products, and those which can only be categorized as 'miscellaneous'. Indeed, the fact that classification of wart treatments poses such difficulties is itself significant; this problem is not encountered when considering the home remedies for any other ailment.

If we consider first the domestic remedies for warts which use plants, we find that the list is a remarkably long one. Rather than listing the species, these are summarized in Appendix I. It will be seen from this summary that over forty species of plants have been recorded for this purpose. Certainly further studies would reveal even more. Among the commonest of plant cures for warts in Britain are dandelion juice (*Taraxacum officinale*) spurge juice (*Euphorbia* spp.) and the juice of greater celandine (*Chelidonium majus*, a member of the poppy family, not to be confused with the lesser celandine). In these three cases the juice of the plant is rubbed on to the wart and allowed to dry. Petty spurge (*Euphorbia peplus*) is known in Cornwall as wartweed, while another species of spurge, sun spurge (*Euphorbia helioscopia*) was known in Orkney as warty-girse.[1] Rubbing with the inner fluffy lining of a broad bean pod is another very commonly reported treatment for warts.[2] After repeated applications, the wart shrivels and disappears. These, and some of the other plant cures for warts, appear to be the typical common-sense first aid applied by country people to so many ailments. No particular ritual is involved. Numerous other plant juices, such as St John's wort (*Hypericum* sp.), milkwort (*Polygala* sp.), sow thistle (*Sonchus arvensis*), potato (*Solanum tuberosum*), fig (*Ficus carica*), pineapple (*Ananas comosus*) are used similarly.

However, there are a number of plant remedies, including apple (*Malus domestica*) and the sloe (fruit of blackthorn, *Prunus spinosa*), which have an accompanying ritual when they are used for wart treatment. The apple is cut in half, rubbed on the wart, and then buried in the ground.[3] The theory is that as it rots, the wart will disappear. The sloe is cut, rubbed on the wart and thrown over the left shoulder.[4] These remedies seem to occupy an intermediate position between the purely common-sense remedy, such as dandelion juice, and the fantastical ones described below. A remedy recorded from Ireland involved touching the warts with nine blades of timothy grass (*Phleum pratense*), while a prayer was said;[5] here evidently the plant itself was of secondary importance. Other cures involve cutting notches in an elder stick equal in number to the warts, or pricking as many holes as there are warts in an ivy leaf.[6] Again, in these two cures, the actual plant used seems to be relatively unimportant. An author on Calendar Customs in Ireland tells us that 'It was firmly believed that any herb picked at random before sunrise on Mayday was an infallible cure for warts'.[7] In this instance there can be no doubt that the ritual is more important than the plant ingredient itself. There is thus a gradation in plant remedies for warts, from those that are purely empirical, to those that are magical.

Presumably the wide variety of wart cures still in existence, many of them with a ritualistic element, reflects an early observation that warts can mysteriously appear and disappear. The appeal of magic is strong, even in this day and age; and certainly many wart cures appear to be magic; in other words, we do not understand how they work. Perhaps warts, which do not represent a life-threatening condition, were an area in which imagination was given free rein. This could explain why even some of the plant remedies used in self-treatment of warts have a touch of accompanying magic.

On the whole, though, it is noticeable that wart remedies using plants are apparently more 'sensible' and down-to-earth than those using other ingredients. Of the

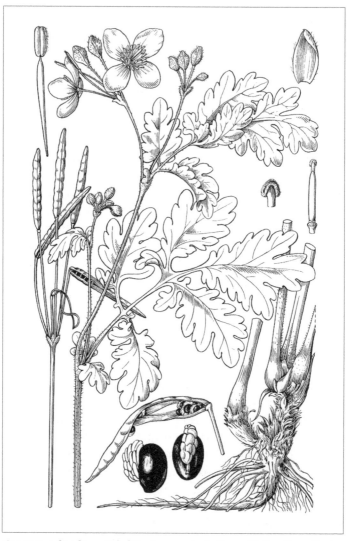

Greater celandine (*Chelidonium majus*), from Stella Ross-Craig, *Drawings of British Plants*. (By kind permission of the Royal Botanical Gardens, Kew/photograph courtesy of John Innes Foundation Historical Collections)

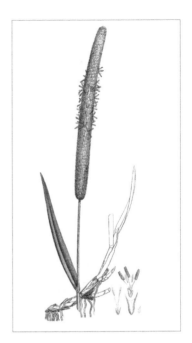

Timothy grass (*Phleum pratense*), from Sowerby's *English Botany*. (Photograph courtesy of John Innes Foundation Historical Collections)

few wart-treating plants that have been investigated scientifically, several have been shown to have anti-viral properties,[8] and some are currently being investigated for their possible anti-cancer effects.[9] The scant scientific evidence available suggests that common-sense plant remedies for warts may indeed have been effective for phytochemical reasons, though there is relatively little data available on the detailed plant chemistry of most of the plants traditionally used in wart treatment. Petty spurge (*Euphorbia peplus*), one of many spurges to be used in wart treatment, has recently been shown to contain steroids,[10] while caper spurge (*Euphorbia lathyris*) has yielded an anti-tumour principle.[11] As further information accumulates, it might eventually be possible to assess the effectiveness of traditional plant remedies for warts in terms of their phytochemistry.

As is the case for so many minor ailments, the plants used by official medical herbalists in Britain today are different from those used in home cures. A modern *Encyclopedia of Medicinal Plants* cites the use of *Aloe vera* and of *Thuja occidentalis* (white cedar) in the treatment of warts.[12] Neither of these is a native British plant. It is interesting to note that neither plant figured in a survey of wart cures done in the 1960s:[13] however, a recent survey yielded two records of the use of *Thuja* sp.[14] This presumably reflects the replacement of the country traditions with those of official herbalism. Chevalier refers to the use of *Chelidonium majus* (greater celandine) latex for treatment of warts, and adds that the juice slowly breaks down the warts by the effect of its protein-dissolving enzymes.[15]

Going back further in time, an attempt to trace twentieth-century traditional wart remedies is made extra difficult by the fact that, in the past, the term 'wart' seems to have covered all kinds of skin blemishes, probably including some that were cancerous. Warts, corns and moles were often lumped together. However, it is interesting to find that John Moncrief of Tippermalloch includes in his *Poor Man's Physician* of 1731 the use of burnt willow ashes, the juice of great celidon (*Chelidonium majus*) and the juice of spurge, as well as rubbing with an apple.[16] Willow (*Salix* sp.) is a known source of salicylate, which still today forms the basis of many patent wart medicines. The greater celandine (*Chelidonium majus*), and various spurges (*Euphorbia* spp.), as well as apple juice, have all been recorded in use in the twentieth century: indeed both greater celandine and spurge are still used as home cures for warts today. Despite the superstitions surrounding wart treatment, it seems that the plants themselves were often a practical element. Susan Palliser, in her monograph on plants as wart-cures in seventeenth-

and eighteenth-century England, points out that, even in the case of the magical cures for warts, 'these were generally combined with the practice of rubbing the afflicted area with the sap or juice from a plant'.[17]

It is my impression that wart remedies are not quite as well represented in the traditional remedies of the past as they are in living-memory remedies. Compared to other common ailments, they appear relatively rarely in the diaries and the kitchen books of the seventeenth and eighteenth century; yet when one comes to study living-memory remedies, they are among the commonest. The explanation of this could be simply that in the past they were largely ignored, because they were not regarded as serious or life-threatening in any way; or warts could have been less common than they are today, though this seems unlikely. The preponderance of wart cures in any present-day study of home remedies perhaps reflects the fascination with which we all regard them, which could be the reason why such traditions have survived when other more down-to-earth plant remedies have been forgotten. Indeed, 'wart cures' were the blight of my life when I began to study plant remedies. Repeatedly, when I was hoping to hear about remedies for coughs, colds, cuts, etc., I found myself being told weird and wonderful wart stories instead!

Many traditional treatments for warts do not use plants. Indeed, the list of ingredients even of twentieth-century wart cures reads more like the contents of a Shakespearean witch's brew than anything else. Blood from a mole, menstrual blood, urine, spit, well-water, forge water, white pebbles, red cord; the list is endless. Usually there is some accompanying ritual, often to be performed in secrecy. Rubbing with a piece of fresh meat seems to be a very common 'cure', and in many cases it is specified that the meat should be stolen. Having rubbed the wart, the meat must then be buried in secret. A common East Anglian wart remedy, recorded repeatedly during this century, and used within living memory, is to rub the wart with the belly of a black slug (or more rarely a snail). The unfortunate slug is then to be impaled on a thorn bush and, as it rots, so the wart will vanish. Writers of folklore stress the element of 'transference' of the wart from the sufferer to the object used in treatment.

Interestingly, many wart cures have a built-in time factor: they involve rubbing the wart with a slug, a snail, a piece of stolen meat, etc. The object is then thrown away or buried, and as it rots so the wart will disappear. In the time taken for the object to rot, many warts may well have disappeared without any treatment; they are an example of a self-limiting condition. It is widely recognized in orthodox General Practice that many self-limiting conditions will have righted themselves, with or without treatment, by the time the patient comes for a return visit. Presumably the time clause in many wart cures is a result of the observation that eventually many warts will disappear by themselves.

It is very striking that wart remedies are still very easy to collect, and many are still in current use. A recent survey came up with the surprising finding that almost two-thirds of informants had suffered from warts at some time during their lives.[18] Also of interest is the fact that the majority had tried unorthodox treatment, ranging from rubbing with a piece of stolen meat, to having recourse to a wart charmer. The success rate seems to have been quite high, regardless of the method used. All this suggests either that warts are more susceptible than most ailments to psychotherapy, or else that they resolve themselves without treatment. Whether the treatment helps them on their way is far harder to ascertain! Presumably there is a psychological element involved here. The patient who has no treatment for his or her condition may take longer to get better than the patient given any treatment that is perceived as effective, whether or not it is. A modern analogy would be the patient attending a doctor's surgery with a mild viral infection. The doctor knows that this will probably get better without any treatment, but may advise the use of a tonic, or an appointment for a follow-up visit. Either of these may prove more effective than nothing. It is a well-known observation that warts can spontaneously disappear, so some at least of the successes may have owed nothing to the method used. This does seem to be a field ripe for enquiry.

Increasingly, orthodox medicine is finding links between patient attitudes towards illness and the success of their treatment. This is probably nothing new: our forebears exploited this aspect of the body's own healing powers when they developed healing rituals. It has been suggested in earlier chapters that ritual surrounding plant remedies tended to creep in usually when a healer was involved, rather than in self-treatment. However, in this respect too, warts seem to provide an exception; the ritual seems to be accepted as a part of the wart treatment, even when the treatment is self-administered.

Aside from ritual, it would be inadvisable to dismiss entirely the physical components of some of the more bizarre substances used in wart treatment. Obviously sweat, blood, fresh meat, urine, fasting spittle, and even slugs and snails will contain an enormous variety of ingredients, some of which could have a direct effect on the wart virus. It is possible that the slugs commonly used in East Anglia to treat warts may contain substances that help destroy the wart virus; and the same can be suggested for remedies involving blood, spit, urine, etc. There are numerous records of using saliva to treat warts.

The story of the so-called wart-biter cricket is so strange that one would have believed it belonged to fiction rather than fact. However, the suggestion that it was used as it name suggests is borne out by the fact that it bears this name too in Sweden.[19] There is an analogous record from Norfolk[20] of the use of dragonflies to remove warts:

Old Norfolk Cure
Catch a Dragonfly and holding its wings with thumb and forefinger place it on the hand with the warts. Place the nose of the insect on to each wart when it will gnaw off the offending skin. This process does not hurt and the Dragonfly appears to enjoy the experience. The wart will never grow again.[21]

The animal and mineral ingredients of wart cures are strictly beyond the scope of this book, but a brief list of some of them will highlight their strangeness and diversity. Listeners to a radio programme in the 1960s contributed the following:

rub with cheese or cheese rind;
treat with lime water mixed with cold milk;
or washing soda moistened or dissolved, or with ink;
rub the slime from a small snail on;
steal a piece of meat, rub on wart, then bury meat in the garden – wart will rot as the meat rots;
tie a strand of silk across the wart;
cure dating from Middle Ages – tie piece of horsehair round base of wart;
smear castor oil on wart;
burn the bark from a willow tree, mix ashes with vinegar, apply to wart and leave for twenty-four hours – must be done in secret;

an Old Hampshire cure – moisten good piece of cheddar cheese, roughly size and shape of wart, in the mouth, then flush down the toilet saying 'Wart begone'. Wart will disappear within a week;

rub with a leaf of elder (*sambucus nigra*) while still on the tree, then bury the leaf, all to be done in secrecy;

rub with dandelion juice;

cut an apple in half, eat one half, rub the other on the wart, and then throw over your shoulder, but don't look to see where it goes;

take a pebble from a stream near home, rub it on the wart, then put it in a paper bag and drop it. Whoever picks up the bag is also supposed to take over the wart.

selling warts – 'Give you a penny for your warts'.

One informant stated that hospital treatment for warts had worked, but they returned a year later, and were finally cured using raw beef rubbed on the warts and then buried in the garden. Another had a wart removed with acetic acid, but it always regrew. She found rubbing on a mixture of washing soda and saliva successful.[22] This small selection of wart cures is quite a typical one. Similar cures, with variations, have been recorded from all over the country. In East Anglia, rubbing with stolen beef or bacon seems particularly common, as does the use of a slug or snail.

Apparently even stranger than the slugs and snails is the widespread recourse to wart-charmers, who in most cases seem to have used no agent at all to cure the warts. Often the warts are simply counted, or observed, and the sufferer is told to go home and they will disappear. Often they do. In how many cases would they have disappeared anyway, without recourse to a wart-charmer? This is unanswerable, but it does seem that wart-charming is perceived as effective by its users. The author has spoken to a number of people who recall visiting a wart-charmer with great scepticism, only to find that their warts shortly afterwards disappeared. This would argue against wart charming being entirely a form of faith-healing, since these individuals evidently had no faith at all in the outcome. One individual related how he went in desperation to visit a wart-charmer after all other methods had failed. His job was on the line, as he was a baker's delivery boy and had warts all over his hands. To his own astonishment, the warts vanished shortly after his visit to the wart-charmer.[23] Even more surprisingly, there are several records of animals having their warts charmed away: again, the statistics are not available to prove whether these animals would have recovered equally quickly without a wart-charmer. However, one first-hand story concerns a horse entered for a show that developed unsightly warts just before the show-date. The vet said there was no quick treatment he could provide. A local man with the reputation of being able to charm warts was called. The next day the horse's warts had all gone.[24] The speed of this cure is very hard to dismiss as spontaneous recovery.

There are numerous reports, many of them first-hand, of 'selling' and 'buying' of warts. Usually the healer offered to buy the warts from the sufferer for a small sum. In many instances this seems to have been successful. In the early years of this century, warts, particularly on the hands, seem to have been more common than they are today, a fact that has been remarked by many of my informants. This they variously attribute to improved hygiene, or improved diet.

A remarkable story was told to me by a retired Norfolk schoolteacher. A visitor to the school noticed that one child had particularly nasty warts on his hands, and offered to buy them for a penny. This was done, and the child's warts vanished. Years later, the teacher noticed a child in his own class with warts on his hands. Remembering the visitor from years ago, the teacher decided to try his hand at buying the child's warts. This he did, again for a penny. The child's warts disappeared, but a week or so later, the teacher noticed a wart on his own hand, the first he had ever had! He could not get rid of it, and had it burnt off at the hospital with liquid nitrogen![25]

In a letter written to Mark Taylor in the 1920s there is the following account of a well-known local wart-charmer. It is typical of many such accounts:

> For years there was an old lame man in Heacham named Tom Cooper, who had inherited the 'gift' from his father and grandfather, and his stories of his and their successful cures were very curious. The father was said to have cured 155 warts on one man. When Tom Cooper became old and feeble he said he felt the 'power' was leaving him, and he told my sister the secret of the remedy, warning her at the same time 'If you ever tell it, the power'll leave you and go to the person you tell it to.' Of course she tried it and had some wonderful cures! – She frankly owns that she can't see why the remedy cures.[26]

In earlier chapters, it has been stressed that plant remedies used in domestic medicine are in general free from accompanying ritual. In this respect, the wart treatments appear to be an outstanding exception. Why this should be the case is difficult to determine; the best explanation seems to be that people must have long ago observed that warts seem to be susceptible to an extraordinary variety of treatments. Perhaps almost anything works, and we have indulged our imagination and liking for magic to invent extraordinary wart-cures? An alternative explanation could be that the warts spontaneously disappear, with or without treatment, and that all the weird and wonderful wart-cures reported are totally irrelevant. Against this argument, there is evidence that treatment seems to trigger recovery more quickly than non-treatment.

There is a third possible explanation. It is possible that warts, more than any other common ailment, are susceptible to *self*-healing, and it is this feature that is being exploited in all the strange wart cures we have invented. We have seen in other chapters how in the traditional treatment of many ailments elements of ritual usually accompany treatment by a healer, rather than self-treatment. Warts could be an exception in this respect because we are tapping into our own powers of self-healing, which in this particular condition have been found to work well. This idea would tie in with the observed success of hypnotherapy in the treatment of warts. An American study showed hypnotherapy to be effective for treating warts in pre-pubertal patients, and for adults when used as an individual hypnoanalytical technique.[27] All the evidence points to a strong 'faith-healing' element in the cure of warts. One lady went to her GP with warts; he assured her that they would be gone in a week, and they were.[28] The family doctor's life would be very easy if all ailments could be cured this easily!

The efficacy of all the wart remedies mentioned so far is extremely difficult to assess; judged by anecdotal evidence, all the methods mentioned have had their measure of success. As regards actual scientific evidence for the possible efficacy of the constituents used, this is sparse for the plant remedies, and almost entirely lacking for the animal and miscellaneous ingredients.

Another possible reason for the diversity and frequency of traditional wart remedies, and for their survival up to the present day, may be the perceived lack of success of orthodox remedies. Most of these involve application of a caustic substance (e.g. salicylate-based), cautery with liquid nitrogen, or surgical removal. All of these methods succeed in some cases, but none appears infallible, so that a recent paper on wart treatment points out 'the search for a reliably effective wart treatment goes on'.[29] An interesting survey of wart patients in the Belfast area shows that among a group of more than 800 patients, nearly one-eighth had used some kind of semi-magical treatment prior to attending the clinic. Obviously in these cases at least the charming was unsuccessful. The author suggests that the dramatic cures sometimes reported are probably the result of the ritual coinciding with the end of the natural life of the wart.[30] This is clearly difficult to prove or disprove.

The oddness of warts and their cures finds reflection in the attitude of the medical profession towards them. Whereas there is rarely an acknowledgement of the traditional remedies for an ailment on the part of British doctors, the medical literature on warts abounds in references to weird and wonderful wart cures. The subject holds a fascination even for the modern orthodox doctor. One dermatologist goes further. At the end of a very interesting and entertaining review of the history and folklore of warts, he has this advice:

If, after spitting toothpaste-free early morning saliva on their warts until blue in the face, slaughtering various small furry and slimy creatures, and spending long, lonely moonlit nights at the cross-roads with hands in a sodden, rotting tree stump waiting for a passing funeral, your patient's warts persist, try giving them a referral letter to the local wart clinic. They don't have to keep the appointment – the author has been told on a number of occasions 'I think I'm wasting your time doctor. As soon as the appointment arrived the warts started to go.' So maybe your local dermatologist has occult powers you never suspected.[31]

In a review published in 1979, an American dermatologist concluded his survey of warts in European medical folklore with these words: 'While science reveals more and more truths to us, many people seem to hold back. They embrace faith and hope and fantasy (which are warmth and softness, love and acceptance) while the world grows cold about them.'[32]

No consideration of the folklore of warts would be complete without reference to the supposed causes of warts. Whereas theories of the origins of many trivial ailments seem not to have occupied the minds of those who used traditional plant remedies, warts in this respect, as in so many, are an exception. Warts have been ascribed to insufficient washing of hands, to washing in water in which potatoes have been cooked, or in which eggs have been boiled. The following extract is from a letter written by a retired Suffolk schoolmaster in the 1960s:

In North Suffolk most children years ago suffered at some time during their life – and adults as well from Warts – chiefly on the hands. Practically all of them called them Wrets or Rets and the word wart was seldom used ... Probably they came because there was not so much washing of the hands as now and particularly among children they have largely disappeared because of the cleanliness insisted in schools.

Why they came was accounted for by a number of reasons. One was that they seeded. Another was that if one was cut and bled and the blood came on another part of the hand, then a ret would come. Another very common belief was that if a person washed his or her hands in water in which eggs had been boiled then warts resulted from this. Another reason given was that they were 'wished' by someone else on you.

I think that the rough dirty work done by most – adult or young in an agricultural district and other rough trades caused them. There were many methods of getting rid of them.

The most common was that in every small town or village there was some person who had the power to get rid of them – mostly a man. According to the man various methods were used. One common one was to get a garden snail, smear the ret with the spit or slime bubbles from the snail on the wart then he would impale the snail on a thorn and the person was warned to forget about it and the wart would waste.

Another was for the man to touch the wart with something after looking at it, say some words, bury the thing and then the wart would gradually fade.[33]

It has been suggested that killing a toad can cause warts. However fanciful these ideas may seem, it should be pointed out that in recognizing the contagious nature of warts, folk medicine was way ahead of the medical profession. Traditional remedies avoided cutting of the wart, which could produce bleeding; presumably this was as a result of the observation that warts could be spread from one person to another or from one part of the body to another. However, it was not until the late nineteenth century that the contagious nature of common warts was clearly recognized by the medical profession.[34]

One last way in which warts prove to be an exception among home-treated ailments is that various plants have been cited as actually *causing* warts. Among these are snowberry (*Symphoricarpos albus*), recorded in Kent in the

1930s as supposedly causing warts; poppy (*Papaver rhoeas*), called wartflower in Cornwall, and reputedly believed in Cornwall to produce warts; and sheep's bit (*Jasione montana*). Picking the flowers of this last species was supposed in Cornwall to give one warts.[35] In all three cases the 'threat' of warts might of course be a way of prohibiting the picking of these flowers, rather than a serious belief that they could cause them.

This is a far from comprehensive account of traditional remedies for warts; however, enough examples have been given to demonstrate that wart remedies differ from the plant remedies used for most minor ailments in one significant respect; they involve ritual and superstition, even though in many instances they are self-administered.

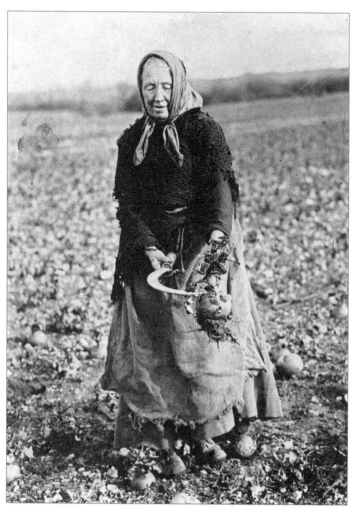

Miss Mary Alcock of Sculthorpe, Fakenham, the oldest member of the Land Army in Norfolk. (From *The Landswoman*, the journal of the Land Army, March 1919. © Norfolk Rural Life Museum)

7

HEDGEROW OR HERB PATCH

Sources of Plants used in Domestic Medicine

Plants used in remedies can be collected in the wild, they can be cultivated, or they can be bought in dried or other preserved state from the chemist or herbalist. The typical, sentimentalized, picture of the herbal user in the past portrays him or her scanning the countryside for the plants needed. In practice, only the paid healer probably spent much time in the gathering of herbs. The use of wild plants in self-treatment was probably limited to the simplest type of remedy. The poorly paid labourer might well use plants in a medical emergency; in the case of a serious cut, for example, he might grab a cobweb and wrap it round the wound,[1] or a puffball (*Lycoperdon* spp.) hanging in the barn might be used to staunch the bleeding.[2] Ivy leaves crushed and placed on a burn is another example of first-aid from the wild. A child with earache might have the juice of a houseleek (*Sempervivum tectorum*) squirted into the ear; the same plant, often to be found growing on the roofs of outhouses, was made into a poultice to treat abscesses and boils.[3]

Among the more leisured classes, the lady of the house might gather a number of plants from the wild, to be made into ointments, etc. In the numerous kitchen books of the wealthy there are frequent references to gathering the necessary plants at their correct time for harvest. Probably only the relatively wealthy could afford the time for such forward planning: certainly only the relatively wealthy have left behind them a written record of their preparation of plant remedies. The sheer quantities involved in some of the more elaborate remedies would suggest that many of the plants involved, even though native to Britain, were deliberately cultivated in the gardens of the wealthy. In the eighteenth-century *Gunton Household Book*, for instance, there is this reference to a Bed of scurvy grass (*Cochlearia* sp.):

A Drink for a Dropsy

Take a quart Bottle, the weight of a Shilling of Horse Raddish and a dozen Raysons stoned and then fill up your bottle with middle beer and stop it then carry it to the scurvy grass bed and put into it leaves, then stop it close and drink it at two days old.[4]

Various species of this plant are common around the coasts of Britain, and were evidently used in the treatment of scurvy.[5] For those living inland, probably only the well-to-do would have enough land and leisure to cultivate this plant. The poor were more likely to have used a more readily available plant, or to have gone without.

The history of the cultivation of plants in many ways mirrors the history of plant medicine itself, and the divergence of folk medicine from orthodox medicine. In Britain, the monks and nuns were early gardeners, as well as early healers, and medicinal and food plants were the most important aspects of their gardens. Initially this was true too for the gardens of the laity, but as gardens gradually became a symbol of gentility, they were used more and more for pleasure, less exclusively for usefulness; eventually, in the nineteenth and early twentieth centuries, medicinal plants were grown little if at all. Now it seems that we have come full circle, and it is again fashionable among the middle classes to cultivate medicinal herbs. However, these medicinal herbs include relatively few of our native British plants. The usage of these has largely been forgotten, simply because they have in the past been mainly used by the silent majority, who have left little or no record of their usage.

The seventeenth-century physician John Pechey in the preface to his *Herbal* states:

> In the first part of the following Herbal, I have only describ'd such Plants as grow in England, and are not commonly known; for I thought it needless to trouble the Reader with the description of those that every Woman knows, or keeps in her Garden.[6]

Pechey's comments were obviously addressed to his literate readers, who would presumably come mostly from the upper echelons of society. Those who relied on domestic medicine during the seventeenth century would include all sectors of society, but the labouring classes would have to depend largely on their own resources, and would not have the benefit of printed books.

The garden of a farm labourer, if indeed he had one at all, would have looked very different from that of a country housewife. The following picture is painted by William Alexander of the typical 'yard' or garden in an Aberdeenshire hamlet in the eighteenth century:

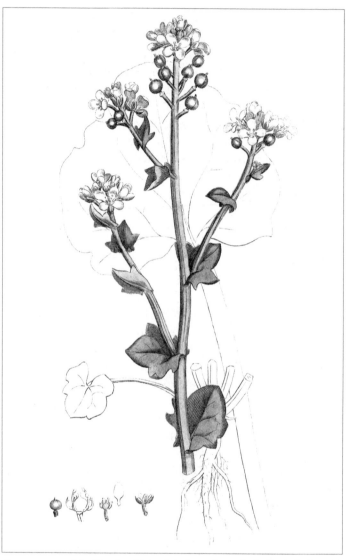

Scurvy grass (*Cochlearia officinalis*), from Sowerby's *English Botany*.
(Photograph courtesy of John Innes Foundation Historical Collections)

About the place we find here and there an exceedingly rustic sort of garden. In these 'yards', which occur in no regular order – are so placed, in fact, that a stranger could hardly guess from the position of any one of them to which of the indwellers it belonged – may be found, besides certain useful vegetables, as 'kail', green or red, and 'syboes', a few old fashioned herbs and flowers. Some clusters of rich-scented honeysuckle, a plant of hardy southernwood, peppermint, and wormwood; with, mayhap, also a slip or two of 'smeird docken', the sovereign virtues of whose smooth green leaves, in respect of sore fingers or broken shins, commend it to careful consideration.[7]

Southernwood (*Artemisia absinthe*), peppermint (*Mentha piperita*) and wormwood (*Artemisia absinthium*) have all been used in the past in traditional domestic medicine, as well as in orthodox medicine and in modern herbalism (see pp. 161, 184). The peppermint referred to here may not be the true peppermint, which was introduced into the official pharmacopoeia early in the eighteenth century, but was initially used mainly in England.[8] However, the book was written by a lawyer, rather than a botanist, and he may well have been referring to any form of mint. As for the 'smeird docken', the botanical identity of this, too, is ambiguous. In the present century, 'smear docken' has been used in Scotland as a name for good King Henry (*Chenopodium bonus-henricus*), which was eaten as a vegetable.[9] However, this plant has rather small leaves, which are not strikingly smooth, and it seems much more likely that Alexander is referring to dock (*Rumex* sp.), all parts of which have been used in traditional medicine. Botanical niceties apart, this description does serve to suggest that the garden of a farm labourer was almost entirely a practical source of food and first aid.

Going further back in time, a similar picture is painted by Tusser for the mid-sixteenth century. At this time, Howe suggests that 'most herb-and-flower plots of the peasant class were maintained on a purely communal basis', and quotes from Tusser:

> Good huswifes in summer will saue their owne seedes,
>> against the next yeere, as occasion needes.
> One seede for another, to make an exchange
>> with fellowlie neighbourhood seemeth not strange.[10]

The impoverished labouring classes had neither the leisure nor the resources for a garden that was purely aesthetic, and the garden, like the rest of their lives, had to pay its way and grow food and medicine. The history of gardens tends to be the history of gardens of the wealthy, in much the same way that the history of herbal medicine tends to be the history of usage of plants by the relatively well-off.

Even the so-called 'cottage garden' has become sentimentalized in Victorian times. Miss Mitford's description of the cottage garden as 'covered with vines, cherry trees, roses, honeysuckles and jessamines, with great clusters of tall hollyhocks running up between them'[11] prompted this bitter response:

> As for hollyoaks at the kitchen doors, and honeysuckles and jasmines,
> you may go and whistle;
> But the tailor's front garden grows two cabbages, a dock, a ha'porth
> of pennyroyal, two dandelions and a thistle[12]

To what extent did people in the past in Britain gather their medicine in the wild, and to what extent did they bring it into their gardens? This would be an interesting idea to explore further, but it is probably very difficult to answer. The fact that traditional plant medicine uses mainly native plants might at first suggest that herbs were generally gathered in the wild, but this was not exclusively so. Possibly a few 'wildings' were cultivated deliberately, as were a few non-native plants (notably houseleek in East Anglia).

The following extract from Mary Webb's book, *The Golden Arrow*, suggests that those with a local reputation as healers did grow many of the plants they used in their garden:

> Her cottage stood among the white mounds, with a strip of garden at the back where she grew her 'yarbs'. Here were horehound, tansy, pennyroyal, balm o' Gilead, all-heal, mallow and a hundred more ... Her acknowledged patients – old folk with rheumatism, rickety children, field workers with a gashed hand or a whitlow, drunkards' wives with bodies covered with bruises – she prescribed for with surprising efficiency; her cures were simple, often drastic, usually very sensible.[13]

Since many of the plants used in traditional medicine were common (and more common in the past than they are now, thanks to urbanization, crop-spraying and pollution), they would probably not be worth the effort of cultivation when used simply as self-medication. Evidence from oral history suggests that gathering in the wild was the commoner picture, at least in situations where the necessary plants were common enough in the wild. In Chapter 4 an account of a 'hermit' who earned a reputation in the Hainault Forest for the ointments he made, mentions that the fern he used was becoming scarce.[14]

Because the poorly paid farm labourer had little time or energy for cultivating a garden, any home remedy, but especially one used in an emergency, would have been of the 'grab-it-and-slap-it-on' variety. The use of a dried puffball for staunching the bleeding of cuts is a good example of this. In the early years of the twentieth century it was common to keep a puff-ball handy in the kitchen or the shed, and it was used for humans and animals alike. And, as mentioned in Chapter 4, other twentieth-century informants have reported using numerous plants such as mallow and elder gathered from the wild.[15] So what determined whether the source of a plant remedy was a wild plant or a deliberately cultivated one? Twentieth-century evidence suggests that the poorer the household, the more likely a plant remedy was to be gathered in the wild: this may simply be a reflection of the lack of garden. The country dweller with a garden could grow much of what was needed. Although the farm labourer probably did not cultivate a purely medicinal garden some of the plants he grew would have been medicinal and he might well have used either these or plants from the hedgerow as remedies.

Tantalizingly, the lack of written evidence means this picture is difficult to establish with certainty. However, if we extrapolate back from twentieth-century evidence, the picture that emerges is of country people using both wild and cultivated plants in times of illness. Doris Coates, in her book *Cottage Housekeeping*, describes self-medication at the beginning of the twentieth century, and tells us that 'Country people felt on safer ground with herbal remedies. Not only were they freely available, but they had an historic use, and previous generations had believed them to be efficacious ... The herb patch was an important corner of the cottage garden.'[16] The author lists, as medicinal plants grown in the cottage garden: balm, betony, camomile, comfrey, golden rod, mallow, rosemary and tansy. She then adds, 'The foregoing herbs were widely cultivated, but many wild plants were highly prized for their curative properties. Here are a few of the simples I remember helping to gather as a child, between 1915 and 1925.' The list includes: eyebright, chickweed, marjoram, meadowsweet, scabious, self-heal, yarrow and yellow loosestrife.

A similar picture of family country medicine composed of plants sometimes gathered in the wild, sometimes grown in the garden, has emerged from the large number of letters I have received. In the following extract is an example of plants used from the garden, which are a mixture of native and non-native species:

My granny had numerous bottles of different tinctures on a sunny windowsill. Unfortunately I remember only a few of them. One was with tincture of arnica (*Arnica montana*). The yellow arnica flowers we picked at roadsides and infused into pure alcohol. We put it on sprains and bruises. Marigold tincture, made from the common marigold flower and alcohol was also used for sprains and for sores. When our cows had sore teats, this remedy cured them.

In another bottle were the flowers of the madonna lily, infused in oil, this tincture was meant to ease burns.

A chamomile tea was used successfully when I had swollen eyes through exposure to reflection of the sun on the snow. The infusion was used to dampen cotton wool pads which were rested on the closed lids for specific periods – very soothing.

When anyone in our family had an upset stomach, they drank vermouth (*Artemisia* sp.) tea made from the vermouth plant which grew in our garden. It tasted very unpleasant.

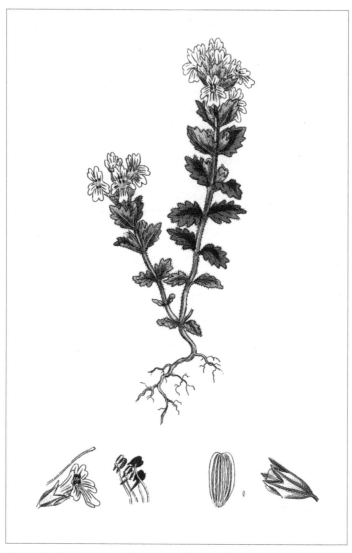

Eyebright (*Euphrasia* sp.), from Sowerby's *English Botany*. (Photograph courtesy of John Innes Foundation Historical Collections)

Groundsel, which can be found almost everywhere in the garden, was used for healing chapped hands. The fresh roots were cut up and simmered in water.

From our home-produced lard my mother used to make hand cream. Lard and elderflowers were simmered together and then strained.

And then there were the various winter remedies: In front of our house stood an old lime tree. It was very big and hollow and we could play 'hide-and-seek' in it. During June we picked the blossoms and dried them in the loft. When someone had flu lime tea was brewed and drunk which made us sweat. This tea was made by pouring boiling water onto the lime blossoms, left for eight minutes and then strained ...

A syrup consisting of very young shoots of the pine trees and sugar, matured on a sunny windowsill, was given to children, when they had a cough. They loved it.

Boiled onions were on the menu when someone had a cold.

For the postman, the chimneysweep and the bellringer there was always a special remedy waiting: Our home-made elderberry liqueur.[17]

Here is a further example of a family who grew medicinal plants in their garden in the 1920s:

My mother and father kept a corner of their large garden to grow a great many herbs – Coltsfoot, Horehound, Hedge Woundwort as well as all the culinary herbs – Rosemary, Parsley, Sage, Mint, Saffron and Comfrey.

A lot of these were used fresh but many were dried for use in winter. Saffron from crocuses was always dried.

My mother's favourite was the Hedge Woundwort and many boils, carbuncles and the like were brought to a head with poultices made from the leaves.

Her soothing drinks, mulled elderberry, mead and honey syrup were to be tasted to be believed.[18]

In the following extract, we read of someone dependent for first aid largely on wild plants, although the lily remedy mentioned is obviously a garden one:

My mother-in-law was a wonderful person, she was married in the last century at the age of twenty. Her husband was nineteen and he worked on a farm earning 10 shillings a week and they lived in a small cottage.

Through the years they had ten children which the Midwife delivered, sometimes in candle-light. Mother never had a doctor, as you had to pay two shillings and sixpence every time he came. All of her children were perfect, brought up in the natural way and she knew how to treat their ailments ... I always wish I had asked he for some of her remedies.

She would go round the hedgerows collecting leaves. She poured boiling water on them and the children would drink the brew. She always kept a jar full of lily leaves soaked in brandy (which was cheap in those days). When my husband was a boy he had to chop the wood for the fires. One day he chopped the top off his thumb. Mother washed it well, then put the piece back on the thumb and bound a lily leaf on. She got a bandage and wrapped it on so securely it had to stay on for a week. When it was taken off the thumb was all healed up and he never had a scar.[19]

Evidence is accumulating, especially from D.E. Allen's work, of a geographical variation in the plant remedies used for a particular ailment, corresponding with the distribution in the wild of a particular plant.[20] This would argue in favour of the majority of plant remedies being prepared from wild specimens, since any plant growing in

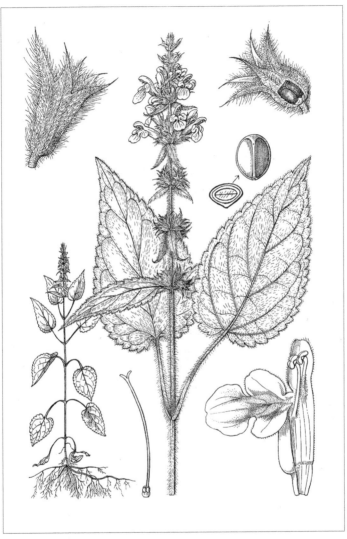

Hedge woundwort (*Stachys sylvatica*), from Stella Ross-Craig, *Drawings of British Plants*. (By kind permission of the Royal Botanical Gardens, Kew/photograph courtesy of John Innes Foundation Historical Collections)

Britain could in theory be cultivated anywhere in Britain. If most medicinal plants used in traditional medicine were grown in gardens, then one would expect to find greater geographical uniformity.

Common sense suggests that there would be no motivation for growing plants that were readily available in the wild; this would be true at least for the rural population, who spent most of their lives out of doors anyway. As wild plants have become rarer and more polluted, it would seem that the picture has altered and, by the beginning of the twentieth century, many plants that could have been freely gathered in the past in the wild were now available mainly as weeds of cultivated land. One informant reported that her aunt insisted on a patch of broad-leaved plantains being preserved in the garden, because she used the leaves for the treatment of varicose ulcers.[21] Some plants, for example many spurges, have become naturalized as weeds in our gardens, and these find use in current domestic medicine (e.g. spurges for warts, ditto greater celandine); so the line between wild and cultivated begins to break down; comfrey, for example, is often naturalized in hedgerows, as a remnant of earlier cultivation. The same is true of feverfew; until the present vogue for its use in migraine, no one deliberately cultivated it, because it appears frequently as a weed of cultivated land.

For the wealthy rural population, such as the lady of a country house, a wide range of both wild and cultivated plants would be available, and the study of seventeenth- and eighteenth-century kitchen books shows that, as one would expect, the home recipes used in domestic medicine are correspondingly more complicated. Of course, it must be borne in mind that we do not have the equivalent written record for the poorer rural population. As discussed in earlier chapters, it appears that ordinary people used mainly 'simples' in their domestic medicine, that is to say single plants, which were generally wild or very easily cultivated. The more complex remedies such as the one given below were probably derived originally from written as well as oral sources; apart from anything else, they would be difficult to remember, which would immediately suggest that they were not used by the illiterate. The following example of a family remedy handed down through generations of a Wiltshire family is a fascinating one. It has survived in written form in a collection of otherwise culinary recipes. The present informant remembers her aunt using this ointment, which was well known in the family as grandmother's ointment:

Burn and Scald ointment
2lbs mutton or deerfat
3 ozs Bees wax
1/2 pt salad oil
2 handfulls Elderflowers gathered fresh
2 handfulls of the inner bark of the Elder
2 Handfulls of the inner bark of the Elm
2 dozen young green ivy leaves
2 handfulls of laurel leaves
2 handfulls of the harts tongue fern
2 handfulls of Houseleek
2 handfulls of Pennywort
2 handfulls of Wild Geranium (Herb Robert)
2 handfulls of Scrophularia (Figwort)
Boil this very slowly together in just enough water to cover it for a long time, then strain it through muslin, it must be well mixed and melted together in the oven before it is potted and tied down it will keep for years and is excellent for Burns, Broken chilblains or any kind of sores.[22]

What are the sources of this recipe? This is probably impossible to answer, but it may well be based on several sources. There is an interesting contrast between this Wiltshire recipe, still used in the twentieth century, and the remedy for burns known to have been used in Ayrshire within living memory, which consisted simply of freshly gathered ivy leaves crushed in oil.[23] Indeed, as far back as the Leechbook of Bald, ivy twigs steeped in melted butter were recommended for sunburn.[24]

Unfortunately, so few of the remedies used by poorer country people have survived that it is not possible to generalize; however, this could be an example of the difference between the simple plant remedy of the poor and the much more complex remedy derived by the literate from all kinds of sources, including folk medicine. Obviously, the leisure to prepare and keep a stock of ointment for a particular ailment would be a privilege of those wealthier than the farm labourer.

There could be another explanation for the evolution of the more complicated plant remedies. It is possible that where someone became known as an expert in treating a certain condition, there would be a tendency for any treatment used to become complicated, in order to distinguish it from the kind of 'simple' that was common knowledge. Tormentil (*Potentilla erecta*) is a common plant of heath and dry pasture, and has been used for centuries to treat diarrhoea, as well as in treatment of wounds and as a gargle. In *Notes and Queries*, 1905–15, there is a report of a Norfolk man over eighty years old, gathering what he called 'a little tormenter' for his wife.[25] Evidently the virtues of this plant were well-known in country areas until recent times:

Thornton tells of a poor old man who made wonderful cures of ague, smallpox, whooping cough, etc., from an infusion of this herb and became so celebrated locally that

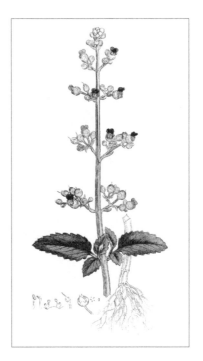

Figwort (*Scrophularia* sp.), from Sowerby's *English Botany*. (Photograph courtesy of John Innes Foundation Historical Collections)

Lord William Russell gave him a piece of ground in which to cultivate it, which he did, keeping it a secret for long.[26]

Now there would have been no need for secrecy had the use of tormentil not been already widespread. One could argue that an alternative approach would have been to make a more complicated remedy involving a number of plants, including tormentil. This could have been the way in which more complex remedies, such as the burn ointment quoted above, came into existence.

Another handed-down recipe, revealed in a collection edited by Brian Friel, is for a remedy used within living memory in Ireland for treating erysipelas. It was composed of the following herbs: daisy (*Bellis perennis*),

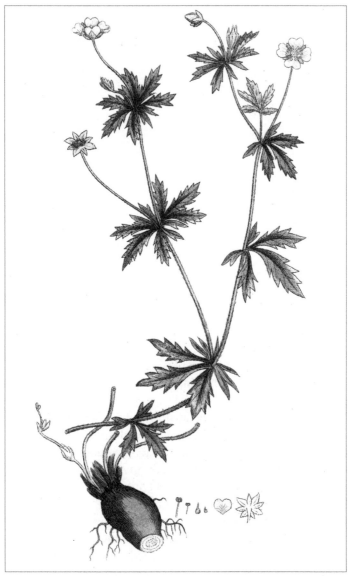

Tormentil (*Potentilla erecta*), from Sowerby's *English Botany*.
(Photograph courtesy of John Innes Foundation Historical Collections)

'stinking roger' (*Scrophularia* sp.) fern, dock, primrose, woodbine (*Lonicera periclymenum*) and pennywort (*Hydrocotyle vulgaris*). The herbs were all ground together in a pot and then applied as a poultice. Was it written down, or purely oral? It would be fascinating to know. Although it belonged strictly to traditional medicine, we are told that, 'Dr Thompson, nephew of Rev Thompson, had great belief in the cure and had all the herbs growing in his garden.'[27] The great majority of herbal remedies mentioned in this fascinating book are single-plant remedies, with no one individual especially associated with them. The 'multiplant' remedy does seem to be the exception rather than the rule among plant remedies used in self-medication.

There are several books of plant remedies written in the twentieth century but based upon the knowledge of an earlier member of the author's family. These books can give us an insight into otherwise unrecorded country medicine. One such is *Mrs Lavender's Herbal Book*, which has no date, but was evidently published between the two World Wars. In the introduction, the author tells us:

> A very wise woman was my grandmother ... I am an old woman myself, well over seventy, though people say I don't look it, my eyes are so bright and my skin is so clear, thanks to my garden; ... grannie must have been about ninety when I was a baby ... and when I was a child she took me round her garden many a day, stopping to gather this sprig or flower or leaf, and telling me how the good God had made them grow that man might make use of them and draw health – yes, and beauty too – from the earth.[28]

The majority of the remedies contained in this book are made from a single common plant, such as dandelion,

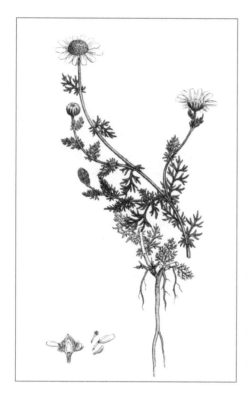

Chamomile
(*Chamaemelum nobile*),
from Sowerby's
English Botany.
(Photograph courtesy
of John Innes
Foundation Historical
Collections)

nettle, dock, alder, chamomile, etc., and presumably they represent the kind of simples used nearly two hundred years ago, when Mrs Lavender's grandmother was a young woman.

These examples provide a picture of native British plants used by rich and poor alike in the country. Those with gardens may have cultivated them, those without collected them in the wild. To what extent was fresh plant material used? Pharmacologically this is of great importance; the effect of a fresh plant extract is often totally different from the effect of an infusion of a dried plant, or an ointment prepared from a fresh or dry plant. The farm labourer would not have time to prepare an elaborate medicine; he was more likely to use the whole fresh plant as a poultice.[29] Ironically, this might have meant that at least some of his home remedies were more effective than the rich man's counterpart, or the urban equivalent. What is clearly illustrated, however, is the wide range of sources from which people – whether rich or poor – obtained the plants for the domestic medicine used in their daily lives.

8

OLD CURES, NEW HEALING

The Effectiveness of Plant Remedies

This enormous and complex subject cannot be exhaustively covered here, but a few points will illustrate the difficulties encountered in any attempt to assess the efficacy of a historical plant remedy. For a start, there is rarely any direct evidence one way or another as to whether a particular remedy was found to be effective. One therefore has to rely on speculative argument: would a particular remedy persist over a widespread area and for a long time if it were not effective? Perhaps it would if no better alternative were available. On the other hand, one could argue that such remedies have been 'screened' over the centuries, and only the best have been preserved: they have, in effect, been subject to a very long empirical trial (see p. 135). One might expect that some at least of the most persistent and widespread plant remedies were genuinely helpful.

If one assumes that the plant actually used in a historical remedy can be identified correctly in modern terms (and this is a big assumption), then how can we assess its efficacy? Any given plant contains thousands of compounds, any of which, alone or in combination, might be responsible for a therapeutic effect. Identifying a so-called 'active ingredient' can prove almost impossible. However, the problems do not end here. If we assume (another enormous assumption!) that we can identify an 'active principle' in the plant used in a particular remedy, we are still a long way from assessing the efficacy of the remedy.

The factors affecting the biological activity of plant compounds are numerous. The environment in which the plant has grown affects the concentration of many of its compounds, as does the genotype.[1] The season at which the plant is harvested, and even the exact time of day, affects the pharmacological activity. Different parts of the plant contain widely different concentrations. The method of preparation of the plant profoundly affects the activity of many of its compounds: an obvious example is that boiling any plant destroys much of its vitamin C content. Some active principles are lost in drying, others deteriorate quickly over time: yet others are unstable to the extent that only a fresh plant preparation is effective.

So in order to assess the effectiveness even of a known plant with a known clinical activity, we still need to know where the plant was grown, to what genotype it belongs, what part of the plant was used, at what time it was harvested and exactly how it was prepared for use as a remedy. In addition, we need to know the dose given, the body weight of the patient, the number of times it was used, and the time period over which it was used. If all these factors were known (and clearly they never are when we are talking about a historical remedy) then it might be possible to make an objective assessment of the effectiveness of the remedy. But the difficulties do not end here! Every individual varies in his response to a given treatment: what is effective for one may be less so for another.

It is clear that the difficulties in establishing objective efficacy of a particular historical plant remedy are formidable. Nevertheless there is undoubtedly very valuable information to be gleaned from the country remedies of the past and present. Many people know the story of digoxin, extracted from foxgloves, and opiates from the opium poppy. Other recent examples of plant remedies 'vindicated' by modern science include the development of the vinca-alkaloids, used successfully in treating childhood leukaemia, from periwinkle plants (*Vinca* sp.) and the use of extracts of yew (*Taxus baccata*) in treating ovarian cancer. Hypericin from St John's wort (*Hypericum perforatum*) is being investigated for its anti-HIV activity. Undoubtedly there are other valuable remedies waiting to be rediscovered. But in recording the plant remedies used by our ancestors, we must bear in mind all the above caveats before claiming that they were probably effective.

Riddle has recorded an extensive and fascinating collection of plant remedies used in the distant and recent past for abortion and contraception.[2] There is a temptation to claim efficacy for herbs with a known contraceptive activity in those instances where birth rate was known to be low. However, many other factors could have produced the same effect, such as changes in diet or climate. It is true that a study of abortive herbs has the advantage that it is sometimes possible to record the outcome! As Riddle has pointed out, there is a clear-cut result; the pregnancy continues or aborts. But all too often the outcome is not actually recorded. A rare instance where it is, is the ballad quoted in Chapter 2, where Queen Mary's lady-in-waiting tried to abort using juniper, but failed, and was executed in the Tolbooth.

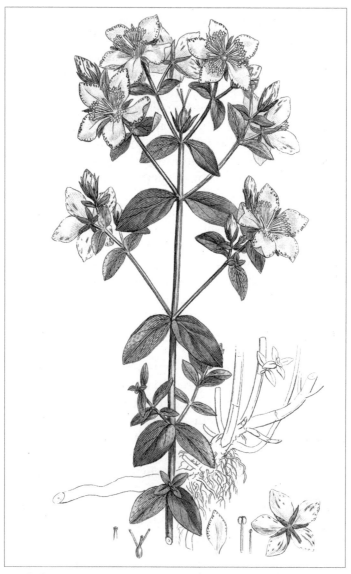

St John's wort (*Hypericum perforatum*), from Sowerby's *English Botany*.
(Photograph courtesy of John Innes Foundation Historical Collections)

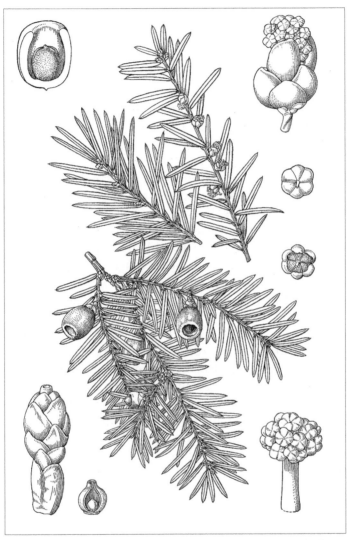

Yew (*Taxus baccata*), from Stella Ross-Craig, *Drawings of British Plants*.
(By kind permission of the Royal Botanical Gardens, Kew/photograph
courtesy of John Innes Foundation Historical Collections)

Another difficulty in attempting to assess efficacy of a plant remedy is that most present-day clinical studies have depended on animal experimentation, or on the use of tissue cultures. One cannot extrapolate reliably from this to the human clinical situation. The story of the acceptance of feverfew as a migraine treatment is a rare example where sufficient human data was available to provide convincing evidence for its efficacy.[3] Subsequent scientific studies of the plant demonstrated both its effectiveness and the way in which it worked.

Until there is some acceptable criterion for assessment of herbal medicines, it is not possible to claim efficacy, especially for a historical remedy. Currently, the Institute of Medical Herbalists, as well as the Institute for Complementary Medicine, are seeking ways in which to evaluate present-day herbal remedies. Even this is very difficult, since herbal medicines do not lend themselves to clinical trial, the tool accepted by the medical profession to study efficacy of a given treatment. Clinical trials depend upon standardization of dosage, route of administration, etc., factors which cannot be standardized in trials of herbal medicines involving plants whose biochemistry is still largely unknown. This difficulty in assessing present-day herbal medicines confirms the impossibility of generalizing about the objective efficacy of plant remedies in the past. This is not to imply that there is nothing of clinical value to be learnt from such remedies. Far from it; much more work is needed in this field. It is important to record all the plant remedies from our past, so as to have a reservoir of information to study in the future. This is of particular importance in Britain, where the oral tradition of using plant remedies is rapidly disappearing. There can be no doubt that among the historical remedies there are some that will prove of clinical value in the future.

Is objective efficacy the whole story? I think emphatically that it is not. All forms of medicine depend on numerous factors apart from pharmacological activity for their effectiveness. The placebo effect is well known and well documented for numerous medicines, but it is poorly understood. A modern drug is deemed effective only if it shows effects greater than the inactive control. But even the placebo effect is better than nothing! Plant remedies used in the past may not have had the effectiveness of modern target drugs, but in many instances they may have provided comfort, the reassurance of being treated, the tonic value of the plants themselves, as well as some measure of effectiveness against the ailment being treated. These elements are vividly expressed in the following extract, taken from living memories of a woman in Essex, where the point is made that the treatment was more than simply its ingredients:

'Wrap this round your throat my dear,' said my mother handing me a long black woollen stocking.

I was in bed with a very sore throat and feeling very miserable. My chest was then rubbed with goosefat and I had some of my mother's cough sweets. Was it my imagination but I began to feel better right away.

When I look back to that distant past I think what an important part home made remedies meant to country folk. We lived some distance from the town and it was difficult to get the doctor to visit as they had to come by horse and trap.[4]

In other instances, the remedies not only had the reassuring effect of a placebo, but contained active ingredients that have since been confirmed as effective: 'We had never heard of anti-biotics or penicillin but knew that wounds healed well if wrapped in cheesecloth with the mold still adhering'.[5] There are numerous examples of this empirical use of moulds, long before the official arrival of antibiotics.[6]

Although the multiplicity of compounds within a single plant makes the pharmaceutical analysis extremely difficult and expensive, this same multiplicity means that a plant taken for one condition may help another, and this observation has been made by several informants. One lady who was preparing poultices of fresh goosegrass (*Galium aparine*) for the treatment of her husband's skin condition, was surprised to find that her own psoriasis benefited greatly from the contact with the fresh plant juice. This plant is currently used by medical herbalists to treat psoriasis, but the lady in question made this discovery for herself. Another informant told me that a friend of hers worked on a herb farm, in which chamomile was grown commercially. When harvesting the plants, she observed great benefit to her own hands, so much so that she asked the manager of the factory for the leftovers after the oil had been expressed. This she used in self-treatment. Feverfew, which as we have already seen hit the headlines in the treatment of migraine, was found by one Suffolk lady to be helpful in reducing the hot flushes of menopause; this information she spread among her friends. A lady in Essex told of an ointment prepared for her husband, under the direction of a local gypsy. It was so dramatic in curing the boils that had cost him his job that she always made up a batch each year. She found it extremely effective in treating chapped hands. Another lady, this time in Norfolk, told of the acute dermatitis suffered by her uncle, which was cured by means of an ointment prepared from dock root. Again, the results were so impressive that she made a jar annually, and found it to be effective in the treatment of all kinds of rashes, including the itchy rash babies suffer after vaccinations. These examples illustrate one way in which the multi-use of a plant for a large number of remedies could have evolved, and Mrs E.M. puts this point vividly: 'Nettle tea we had to drink to purify our blood, Grandpa (unwillingly) for his sciatica and Aunt Rose for her pleurisy. I wondered how it knew which it was supposed to do.'[7]

These anecdotal pieces of evidence show that some plant remedies are effective at least as far as their users are concerned. Probably a similar picture held true in the past. Simple country remedies were used for lack of anything else, and at least in some cases they were perceived as effective. Statistical data is not available to convince the modern clinician, but we surely must conclude that many country remedies did at least some good, and that we would be wise to investigate many of them further.

Although much is said and written about the disappearing rainforest, and the consequent loss of potential medical knowledge, it is not generally appreciated that in Britain we have our own endangered heritage of country knowledge of plants. This knowledge will die out with the last generation of country people to have used it. There is an urgent need to record such knowledge for posterity, as it is a strand of knowledge quite separate from official medical herbalism. The latter owes much to the North American traditions of herbalism, and even in instances where native British plants are used, they are not necessarily used in the same way, or even for the same ailments.

In country medicine, fresh plant material is often used, either simply as juice squeezed out of the plant or in the form of a poultice. It is now known that the chemical properties of fresh plant extracts can sometimes be quite different from those of a dried plant extract. Sometimes

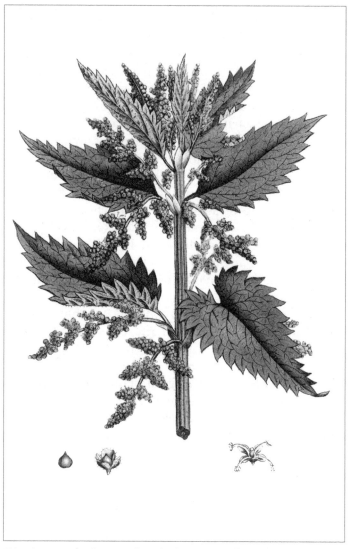

Stinging nettle (*Urtica dioica*), from Sowerby's *English Botany*.
(Photograph courtesy of John Innes Foundation Historical Collections)

the roots and shoots and flowers of one plant species all have different medicinal properties, some of which have been exploited in traditional medicine, but are now largely forgotten by official herbalism.

Currently all forms of complementary medicine are enjoying an upsurge of interest in this country, and medical herbalism is no exception. It is vitally important to take advantage of this interest to combine the best of the country knowledge of the past with the best science of the present. With the backing of such departments as the Centre for Economic Botany at the Royal Botanic Gardens, Kew, it is hoped that British ethnobotany is about to take the place it deserves.

A joint project, called Ethnomedica, has begun, involving medical herbalists and botanists (myself included), with the aim of gathering information about country remedies throughout Britain. At the present time more than forty individual medical herbalists are starting the search in their own localities for knowledge of the country uses of British plants in medicine. Some very interesting information has already come to light. Ironically, this project, at the moment in its infancy, is proving very difficult to fund, probably more difficult than a study involving exotic rainforest plants. But surely in the quest for improved treatments, we should begin in our own back yard!

During the years before the First World War, and during the Second World War, Britain grew large quantities of its own medicinal plants.[8] In addition, a significant quantity of herbs were still gathered from the wild for commercial use. In the *East Anglian Magazine*, December 1972, there is a fascinating account of Cecil Grimes of Wisbech, one of the last men to gather wild plants for a living.[9] As recently as 1962, Cecil was the boss man of the local root diggers:

His gang of diggers ranged far and wide in the East Anglian countryside. They travelled into Essex, Suffolk, Norfolk and Cambridgeshire; the search was often extended to include the countryside of Northampton and Lincolnshire. They dug along the forgotten green roads ... they dug in the green alleys of the fruit orchards ... the roots that were gathered were dandelion, docks, comfrey, mandrake and horseradish ... Dock roots were dried and ground into cures for blood disorders, comfrey roots made into ointment for the treatment of sprained joints and the treatment of open wounds. Dandelion was used for purification of the blood and to restore the loss of appetite. Mandrake was not used for human cures but was sold to farmers and veterinaries for the treatment of sick farm stock ...

During the reign of Elizabeth the First, it would appear the age old right to gather roots was threatened. To preserve the right an act was passed, known as the 'Wild Herb Act', which gave men the right to gather herbs and roots in the wild uncultivated lands. Up to this [twentieth] century the diggers have maintained that they were protected by this legislation to dig for roots in the lanes and hedgerows. Whenever possible they have sought permission to dig upon private land.

Sometimes disputes have arisen, but mostly the farmers are glad to be rid of the so-called weeds and welcomed the root diggers. Then in the year 1962 the men who dried and ground the roots went out of business. The demand was no longer there and the root diggers went out of business.

In East Anglia there was a special 'green herb rate' for sacks of herbs gathered in the wild to be transported by train. Nowadays, even dandelion roots (used by herbalists as a liver tonic and diuretic) are imported from the continent!

However, coinciding with the renewed interest in complementary medicine is the move towards organically grown crops, and towards 'alternative' crops. Firms such as Hambleden Herbs, one of the largest suppliers to Medical Herbalists, are growing an increasing number of herbs, all organically grown. In East Anglia a co-operative of farmers has started to grow, organically, a number of medicinal plants such as marigold (*Calendula officinalis*) and St John's wort (*Hypericum perforatum*).[10] It is hoped that this range will be extended in the near future and, having first determined the optimal growing conditions, a number of medicinal plants can then be grown commercially for supply to medical herbalists. This range will include a number of native British plant species that are now too scarce to be collected in the wild. I am involved with the growing in particular of native British plants whose use has declined in offficial herbalism, owing to their unavailability. Their scarcity in the wild makes their cultivation a necessity.

As a result of co-operation between growers, herbalists and botanists there is a very real hope that some of the traditional usages of British plants in herbalism may be restored, so that even though the old ways have given place to new and self-help has yielded to treatment by professionals, at least some of our valuable heritage of plant wisdom will survive for posterity.

Appendix: Plants Used in the Twentieth Century for Treating Warts

This list is not exhaustive; further studies would undoubtedly add to it.

Alder	(*Alnus glutinosa*)
Apple	(*Malus pumila*)
Ash	(*Fraxinus excelsior*)
Banana	(*Musa* spp.)
Broad Bean	(*Vicia faba*)
Broom	(*Cytisus scoparius*)
Cabbage	(*Brassica oleracea*)
Carrot	(*Daucus carota*)
Castor oil	(*Ricinus communis*)
'Corn' probably wheat	(*Triticum aestivum*)
Chickweed	(*Stellaria media*)
Crowfoot	(*Ranunculus* sp.)
Dandelion	(*Taraxacum officinale*)
Dog's Mercury	(*Mercurialis perennis*)

Elder	(*Sambucus nigra*)
Fig	(*Ficus carica*)
Garlic	(*Allium sativum*)
Greater Celandine	(*Chelidonium majus*)
Ground Elder	(*Aegopodium podagraria*)
Hogweed	(*Heracleum spondylium*)
Houseleek	(*Sempervivum tectorum*)
Ivy	(*Hedera helix*)
Lagwort	(*Petasites hybridus*)
Lemon	(*Citrus limon*)
Marigold	(*Calendula officinalis*)
Milkweed	(? *Silybum marianum*)
Milkwort	(*Polygala* spp.)
Olive oil	(*Olea europaea*)
Onion	(*Allium cepa*)
Pennywort	(*Umbilicus rupestris*)
Poppy	(*Papaver rhoeas*)
Potato	(*Solanum tuberosum*)
Radish	(*Raphanus sativus*)
St John's Wort	(*Hypericum* spp.)
Sloe, fruit of blackthorn	(*Prunus spinosa*)
Sow Thistle	(*Sonchus oleraceus*)
Spurge, Wartweed	(*Euphorbia* spp.)
Stonewort	(Non-flowering plant belonging to Charophyta)
Sundew	(*Drosera rotundifolia*)
Tea-tree	(*Leptospermum* spp.)
Thuja	(*Thuja* sp.)
Timothy Grass	(*Phleum pratense*)
Tobacco	(*Nicotiana tabacum*)
Walnut	(*Juglans* spp.)
Willow	(*Salix* spp.)

NOTES

Introduction

1. W.G. Black, *Folk-Medicine; A Chapter in the History of Culture* (London, Folklore Society, 1883).

Chapter 1: Plant Medicine in Britain

1. Arthur Stanley Broome, *Bob's Boy. Life Story of a Norfolk Countryman*, ed. David Poole (Norwich, Wilson-Poole, 1984), p. 15.
2. J.G., personal communication (Whissonsett, Norfolk, 1988).
3. George Ewart Evans, *The Pattern under the Plough* (London, Faber & Faber, 1966), p. 240.
4. Jonathan Mardle, *Norfolk Characters* (Norwich, George Nobbs, 1976), p. 57.
5. Work done by Alison Cronin at Monkey World, Dorset, reported in *The Week* (September 1998, Issue 172), p. 172.
6. Dr N. Gunn, *The Book of Linton Church* (Peebles, Neidpath Press, 1912), p. 84.
7. Clifford Geertz, *Local Knowledge* (London, Hutchinson, 1993), p. 10.

8.   Ibid., p. 11.
9.   Quoted ibid., p. 80.
10. See for example W. Coles, *Adam in Eden* (J. Streater for Nathaniel Brooke, London, 1657).
11. J.C., personal communication (Hemblington, Norfolk, 1989).
12. Oliver Wendell Holmes, quoted in Mrs C.F. Leyel, *The Magic of Herbs* (London, Jonathan Cape, 1926), p. 253.
13. *Gunton Household Book* (Norwich, Church of St Peter Mancroft).
14. Clerk of Penicuik Papers (Scottish Records Office, GD18 21250).
15. B. Griggs, *Green Pharmacy* (London, Jill Norman and Hobhouse Ltd, 1981).
16. Frank McH., personal communication (1994).
17. See for example Andrew Chevalier, *The Encyclopedia of Medicinal Plants* (London, Dorling Kindersley, 1996), p. 286.
18. Roy Porter, *England in the Eighteenth Century* (London, Folio Society, 1998), p. 15.
19. Tom Higdon, 'The Labourer', quoted in *The Burston Rebellion* (Betka Zamoyska, BBC, 1985).
20. Juliet Gardiner and Neil Wenborn (eds), *British History* (London, Collins and Brown, 1995), p. 14.
21. E.P. Thompson, *Customs in Common* (Harmondsworth, Penguin, 1993), p. 17.
22. Phythian-Adams, C., *Rural Culture*, pp. 623–4 quoted by W.A. Armstrong, in F.M.L. Thompson (ed.), *The Cambridge Social History of Britain 1750-1950*, vol. 1 (Cambridge University Press, 1990), p. 129.
23. National Library of Scotland, MS 3774.
24. S.W.F. Holloway, 'The Orthodox Fringe: The Origins of the Pharmaceutical Society of Great Britain', in W.F. Bynum and R. Porter (eds), *Medical Fringe and Medical Orthodoxy 1750–1850* (London, Croom Helm, 1986), p. 154.
25. J. Young, *Farming in East Anglia* (London, David Rendel, 1967), p.19.
26. E.L.A., d.o.b. 1915, unpublished Age Concern essay (Essex, 1990).
27. D.C.H., d.o.b. 1926, unpublished Age Concern Essay, (Essex, 1990).
28. Mrs B., personal communication (Tacolneston, Norfolk, 1988).
29. Mark Taylor MS (Norfolk Records Office, MS 4322; collected from Wilby Women's Institute).
30. Mark Taylor, see n. 29, Huntingfield Women's Institute.

31. Mark Taylor, see n. 29, informant Baconsthorpe Women's Institute.
32. Mark Taylor, see n. 29, informant Dr Ball, Lowestoft.
33. 'Secenction' is probably ascension weed, or sesension, a local name for groundsel, *Senecio vulgaris*.
34. Lilias Rider Haggard (ed.), *I Walked by Night* (Woodbridge, Boydell Press, 1974), p. 16.
35. See Jacques Rousseau, *Essays in Biohistory* (Utrecht, Netherlands, International Association for Plant Taxonomy, Dec. 1970), p. 195.
36. D.E. Allen, MS.
37. Mrs E.M., d.o.b. 1917, Age Concern essay (Essex, 1991).
38. Mrs E.M., see n. 37.
39. J.A.L, d.o.b. *c.*1930, personal communication (Norwich, 1989).
40. Mrs D.B., d.o.b. *c.*1930, personal communication (Norfolk, 1988).
41. Mr A.E.R., born Essex, d.o.b. *c.*1910, personal communication (Northampton, 1985).
42. Letter from E.J., Co. Mayo, to R. Vickery, 1983.
43. Age Concern Essay, Essex, 1991. Average age of informants eighty years.
44. John M. Riddle, *Eve's Herbs: A History of Contraception and Abortion in the West* (Harvard University Press, 1997).
45. English Folklore Society, record no. 100 (University College London, unpublished).
46. William Buchan, *Domestic Medicine: or a Treatise on the Prevention and Cure of Diseases by Regimen and Simple Medicines* (Glasgow, 1806), p. 605.
47. Joan Perkin, *Victorian Women* (London, Murray, 1993), p. 70.
48. Andrew Chevalier, *The Encyclopedia of Medicinal Plants* (London, Dorling Kindersley, 1996), p. 169.
49. *British Pharmaceutical Codex, 1923* (London, Pharmaceutical Press, 1923), p. 1001.
50. C.P. Petch and E.L. Swann, *Flora of Norfolk* (Norwich, Jarrold, 1968), p. 163.
51. Mary Webb, *The Golden Arrow* (London, Jonathan Cape, 1916), p. 176.
52. Riddle, *Eve's Herbs*, p. 257.
53. P.H. Emerson, *Pictures of East Anglian Life* (London, Sampson Low Marston Searle & Rittington, 1888), p. 91.
54. A.S. Harvey, *Ballads, Songs and Rhymes of East Anglia* (Norwich, Jarrold, 1936).

55. Mary Grieve, *A Modern Herbal* (London, Jonathan Cape, 1931),
     p. 814.
56. Riddle, *Eve's Herbs*, p. 254.

Chapter 2:What Do We Know about Country Remedies?

1.   Clerk of Penicuik Papers, Scottish Records Office, GD 18/2142.
2.   *Gunton Household Book* (Norwich, Church of St Peter Mancroft).
3.   Broughton Cally Papers, Scottish Records Office, GD 10/911.
4.   Clerk of Penicuik Papers, Scottish Records Office, GD 18/2142.
5.   *Gunton Household Book* (Norwich, Church of St Peter Mancroft).
6.   Recipe book of Maryanne Weston of Thorpe, 1825–1884
     (Norfolk Records Office, MC 43/9).
7.   Papers of the Carleton family of Norwich, 1772–*c*.1914, Norfolk
     Records Office, MC 181/82.
8.   George Ewart Evans, *The Horse in the Furrow* (London, Faber &
     Faber, 1960), p. 231 ff.
9.   Mark Taylor, MS (Norfolk Records Office, MS 4322).
10. *Kingsbury Notebook* (Norfolk, Gressenhall Museum, G7.983
     c.1710).
11. Mrs B., Brundall, personal communication (Norfolk, 1988).
12. Mr W.G., personal communication (Witton, Norfolk, 1988).
13. Arthur Stanley Broome, *Bob's Boy. Life Story of a Norfolk
     Countryman*, ed. David Poole (Wilson-Poole, 1984), p. 24.
14. Clerk of Penicuik Papers (Scottish Records Office, GD18/5219),
     quoted in Rosalind K. Marshall, *Childhood in Seventeenth Century
     Scotland* (Trustees of the National Galleries of Scotland, 1976),
     p. 22.
15. Clerk of Penicuik Papers (Scottish Records Office, GD18 2125).
16. John Pechey, *The Compleat Herbal of Physical Plants* (London,
     College of Physicians, 1694), p. 10.
17. Ibid., p. 26.
18. Ibid., p. 37.
19. Ibid., p. 60.
20. Ibid., p. 169.
21. A. Lawson, *The Modern Farrier or the Best Mode of Preserving the
     Health and Curing the Disorders of Domestic Animals* (London,
     1842), p. 282.

22. Mrs T., d.o.b. *c.*1910, personal commmunication (Rockland St Mary, Norfolk, 1989).

23. Mrs E., d.o.b. *c.*1950, personal communication (Whissonsett, Norfolk, 1990).

24. Roy Vickery, *A Dictionary of Plant Lore* (Oxford University Press, 1995), p. 229.

25. Richard Pococke, Bishop of Meath, *Tours in Scotland* (1747, 1750, 1760), ed. D.W. Kemp (Edinburgh University Press, Constable for Scottish History Society, 1887), p. 89.

26. See Pennant's *Tour in Scotland* (1769), p. 310; Lightfoot, *Flora Scotica* (London, 1776), pp. 388, 1132; Defoe, *Tour through Great Britain* (1753), vol. iv, p. 273.

27. Mary Beith, *Healing Threads* (Edinburgh, Polygon, 1995), p. 247.

28. Charles Bryant, *Flora Dietetica or History of Esculent Plants* (London, 1783), p. 37.

29. B.A.F. Pigott, *Flowers and Ferns of Cromer and its Neighbourhood* (Norwich, Jarrold, 1882), p. 8.

30. Alexander Pennecuik, *Description of Tweeddale* (Leith, 1815 edition), p. 312ff and footnote 1.

31. A. Pratt, *Wild Flowers* (London, 1898).

32. P.H. Emerson, *Pictures of East Anglian Life* (London, Sampson Low Marston Searle & Rittington, 1888), pp. 15–17, 91.

33. G.M. Trevelyan, *England under the Stuarts* (London, Folio Society, 1946; reprinted 1966), p. 44.

34. J.C. Smith and E. de Selincourt (eds), *Spenser: Complete Poetical Works* (Oxford University Press, 1912), *Faerie Queen* III, ii, 49.

35. 'Medical Botany' or 'History of Plants' in the *Materia Medica* of the London, Edinburgh and Dublin Pharmacopoeias (London, 1819).

36. Spenser, *Faerie Queene* III, V, 32.

37. J.C. Smith and E. de Selincourt (eds), *Spenser: Poetical Works* (Oxford Universiy Press, 1970), p. 704.

38. Mrs M. Grieve, *A Modern Herbal* (London, Jonathan Cape, 1931), p. 105.

39. Ibid., p. 818.

40. See e.g. G.C. Nuttall, *Wild Flowers as they Grow* (London, Waverley Book Co., n.d.) p. 26.

41. A.E., personal communication (Whissonsett, Norfolk, 1989).

42. Francis James Child, 'The Ballad of the Elfin Knight', in *English and Scottish Popular Ballads*, 8 vols (Boston, 1857–9), vol. I, p. 18.

43. Child, 'Ballad of King Estmere', in *Ballads*, vol. II, p. 53.

44. *Oxford Book of English Verse* (Oxford University Press, 1939), p. 741.
45. Vickery, *A Dictionary of Plant Lore*, p. 1.
46. G. Hatfield, *Country Remedies* (Woodbridge, Boydell Press, 1994), p. 115.
47. Quoted in M. Grieve, *A Modern Herbal* (London, Jonathan Cape, 1931), p. 13.
48. Nuttall, *Wild Flowers*, vol. II, p. 46.
49. Vickery, *A Dictionary of Plant Lore*, p. 211.
50. Anon., 'Ballad of the Queen's Marie', *Oxford Book of English Verse*.
51. Child, *Ballads*, vol. III, p. 387.
52. Pechey, *The Compleat Herbal of Physical Plants* (London, 1694), p. 164.
53. John Jamieson, *A Dictionary of the Scottish Language*, 4 vols and Supplement (Edinburgh University Press, 1808).
54. Geoffrey Grigson, *The Englishman's Flora* (London, Phoenix, 1955), p. 24.
55. *Oxford Book of English Verse*, no. 380.
56. Anne Marie Lafonte, *Herbal Folklore* (Bideford, Badger Books, 1984), p. 77.
57. John M. Riddle, *Contraception and Abortion from the Ancient World to the Renaissance* (Harvard University Press, 1992).
58. See e.g. James A. Duke, *The Green Pharmacy* (Pennsylvania, Rodale Press, 1997).
59. C.N. French (ed.), *A Countryman's Day Book* (London, J.M. Dent & Sons, 1929).
60. Yvonne Skargon, *A Calendar of Herbs* (Scolar Press, 1978).
61. J. Aubrey, *The Natural History of Wiltshire*, J. Britton (ed.), (London, 1847), p. 51.
62. Vickery, *A Dictionary of Plant Lore*, p. 306.
63. Mr W. A., personal communication (Trunch, Norfolk, 1989).
64. Brian Bonnard, *Channel Island Plant Lore* (Guernsey Press, 1993), p. 54.
65. Quoted in R.C. Wren, *Potter's New Cyclopaedia of Botanical Drugs and Preparations* (Devon, Health Science Press, 1975), p. 207.
66. Ibid., p. 311.
67. Nuttall, *Wild Flowers*, vol. I, p. 174.
68. Vickery, *A Dictionary of Plant Lore*, p. 336.
69. Nuttall, *Wild Flowers*, vol. VI, p. 8.
70. Hatfield, *Country Remedies*, pp. 29, 59, 89.
71. Nuttall, *Wild Flowers*, vol. VI, p. 120.
72. Vickery, *A Dictionary of Plant Lore*, p. 143.

73. Nuttall, *Wild Flowers*, vol. III, p. 69.

74. Ibid., p. 73.

75. Grigson, *The Englishman's Flora*, p. 366.

76. Tony Hunt, *Popular Medicine in Thirteenth Century Britain* (Cambridge, D.S. Brewer, 1990), p. 416.

77. Grieve, *A Modern Herbal*, p. 206.

78. Tony Hunt, *Plant Names of Medieval England* (Cambridge, Brewer, 1989), pp. 50, 354, 355.

79. Linda E. Voigts, *Anglo-Saxon Plant Remedies and the Anglo-Saxons*, ISIS, 1979 (No. 252), pp. 250–68.

80. Grieve, *A Modern Herbal*, p. 102.

81. Grigson, *The Englishman's Flora*, p. 89.

82. Hunt, *Plant Names*, p. ix, 'The apparent anarchy of Pre-Linnaean nomenclature does not mean that it had no sense'.

83. William T. Stearn, *Botanical Latin* (London, Nelson, 1966), p. 17.

84. Ibid., p. 15.

85. Hunt, *Plant Names*, p. 394.

86. Hunt, *Plant Names*, p. xvii.

87. Wilfrid Blunt, 'Walahrid Strabo', in *The Hortulus of Walahfrid Strabo* (Pittsburgh, Hunt Botanical Library, 1966). Quoted by Linda Voigts in *Anglo-Saxon Plant Remedies and the Anglo-Saxons*, pp. 250–68.

88. A.G. Morton, *History of Botanical Science* (London, Academic Press, 1981), pp. 98, 113.

89. Ibid., p. 95.

90. Hunt, *Plant Names*, p. 17.

91. Arber suggests that 'in practice, the herbals were used only as reference books, from which to learn the healing quality of herbs with whose appearance the reader was already familiar'. Agnes Arber, *Herbals: Their Origin and Evolution* (2nd edition, Cambridge University Press, 1953), p. 146.

92. William Turner: see preface to *The first and second partes of the Herbal ... with the third parte* (1568).

93. William Turner Facsimiles: *Libellus de Re Herbaria* (1538); *The Names of Herbes* (1548) (London, Ray Society, 1965).

94. Nuttall, *Wild Flowers*, vol. V, p. 135.

95. Hunt, *Plant Names*, p. xvii.

96. Andrea Caesalpino of Arezzo, 1519–1603. His work *De Plantis libri* appeared in 1583. He points out that divisions of plants such as vegetables and kinds of grain are based on their usefulness to man rather than resemblances of form. Moreover, he emphasizes that such properties as medicinal virtues are

'accidental' rather than essential qualities of plants, and should not therefore form the basis of classification. See Julius von Sachs, *History of Botany* (translated H.E.F. Garnsey, Oxford, Clarendon Press, 1890).

97. Cole, quoted in Nuttall, *Wild Flowers*, vol. V, p. 144.

98. Carl Linnaeus, *Critica botanica*, no. 229, quoted in Stearn, *Botanical Latin*, p. 282.

99. *International Code of Botanical Nomenclature*, 1961.

100. A.E., personal communication (Whissonsett, Norfolk, 1990).

101. Dafydd Evans, 'The Doctrine of Signatures as the Explanation of some Puzzling Names and Uses of Plants' in R. Vickery, (ed.) *Plant-Lore Studies* (London, Folklore Society, 1984), pp. 66–74.

102. Grigson, *The Englishman's Flora*, pp. 463, 465.

103. J. Stannard, 'Folk Medicine, Philosophy and Medieval Herbalism', *Res publica litterarum*, 3, 1980, pp. 229–36.

104. Hunt, *Plant Names*, p. l: 'The intriguing question of the continuity or discontinuity of medieval and popular names is one that can scarcely be tackled in the present state of plant-name research, but will certainly be an important topic for future researchers working with more extensive materials.'

105. Mrs D.T., d.o.b. *c.*1910, personal communication (Rockland St Mary, Norfolk, 1988); Mr J.B., Essex, d.o.b. *c.*1920, personal communication (1988).

106. Mr A.R., d.o.b. 1900, personal communication (Cambridgeshire, 1986).

107. Mr M. (born Scotland), d.o.b. *c.*1935, personal communication (Wymondham, Norfolk, 1987).

108. Mr A.B., d.o.b. *c.*1915, personal communication (Whissonsett, Norfolk, 1987).

109. Mrs E.M., d.o.b. *c.*1910, personal communication (Essex, 1985).

110. Mr G., Hemsby, d.o.b. *c.*1920, personal communication (Norfolk, 1989).

111. Numerous records, e.g. Mrs P., d.o.b. *c.*1930, personal communication (Norwich, 1988).

112. Mr and Mrs C., personal communication (Coltishall, Norfolk, 1989); Mrs E.I.J., d.o.b. 1912, unpublished essay for Age Concern (Braintree, Essex, 1990).

113. Mr J.A.L., d.o.b. *c.*1925, personal communication (Norwich, 1988).

114. Mr D.E.B., d.o.b. 1925, personal communication (Essex, 1988).

115. Mrs A.W., d.o.b. *c.*1950, personal communication (Norfolk, 1985).

116. Mr M.C., d.o.b. 1935, personal communication (Norfolk, 1988).
117. Mrs M., d.o.b. 1917, unpublished Age Concern Essay (Essex, 1991); Mrs I.H., Norfolk, d.o.b. *c.*1920, personal communication (Norfolk, 1988).
118. Mark Taylor MS (Norfolk Records Office, MS4322).
119. Mrs D.P., d.o.b. *c.*1910, personal communication (Little Topham, Essex, 1990).
120. Miss N. (born Hampshire), d.o.b. 1920, personal communication (Norfolk, 1988).
121. Woolverstone W.I., Suffolk, recorded 1920s by Mark Taylor (Norfolk Records Office, MS4322).
122. Mr R.C., d.o.b. *c.*1930, personal communication (Norfolk, 1989).
123. Miss N. (born Hampshire), d.o.b. 1920, personal communication (Norfolk, 1985). For more details of these and other East Anglian plant remedies, see Hatfield, *Country Remedies*.
124. See Edward M. Croom 'Documenting and Evaluating Herbal Remedies', *Economic Botany*, 37(1), 1983, pp. 13–27.
125. George Ewart Evans, *Where Beards Wag All* (London, Faber & Faber, 1970), p. 18.
126. Letter from Mrs P.S., Northamptonshire, to Roy Vickery, 1996.
127. Letter to Mr B.M., from Mrs W., West Derby, 1985.
128. Letter from Mr H.W., Suffolk, 1985.
129. Mrs F.E.S., personal communication (Cley, Norfolk, 1990).
130. Mr A.E.R. (born Essex), personal communication (Northampton, 1985).
131. Mrs A.M., personal communication (West Yorkshire, 1985).
132. Mr M.G.R., personal communication (Lakenheath, Suffolk, 1990).
133. Mrs D.T., d.o.b. 1908, personal communication (Rockland St Mary, Norwich, 1985).
134. Hatfield, *Country Remedies*, Ch. 3.
135. George Ewart Evans, 'Flesh and Blood Archives: Some Early Experiences', in *Oral History*, p. 3.

Chapter 3: Simple Plant Remedies: Characteristics of Domestic Plant Medicine

1. William Salmon, *The Compleat English Physician: or, The Druggist's Shop Opened* (London, 1693).

2. Dr Speller, writing in 1974, for example, maintains that 'the foxglove story is one of the few instances where a country remedy has proved to contain an active pharmacological substance. Most of them are to be regarded as superstitious and magical, with success by the patient's belief, or by chance, or not at all.' Letter in *Folklore and Customs of Rural England*, by Margaret Baker (Newton Abbott, Devon, David & Charles, 1974), pp. 169–70.

3. Mr A.A., d.o.b. *c.*1910, personal communication (Trunch, Norfolk, 1988).

4. 'A successful Remedy for a kind of Rheumatism ... Take the inward bark (that which grows next the wood) of an elder tree, cut or tear it into small bits ... pour in ... small ale ... stop it well, till the liquor be strong of the infusion.' 1747, Clerk of Penicuik Papers (SRO GD18/2125).

5. B.W., d.o.b. *c.*1935, personal communication (Hindolveston, Norfolk, 1988).

6. Mary Beith, *Healing Threads* (Edinburgh, Polygon, 1995), p. 215.

7. Roy Vickery, *A Dictionary of Plant Lore* (Oxford University Press, 1995), p. 124.

8. Mrs A., d.o.b. *c.*1900, personal communication (Norfolk, 1989).

9. Carol A. Newall, Linda A. Anderson, J. David Phillipson, *Herbal Medicines* (London, Pharmaceutical Press, 1996), p. 5.

10. G.A. Cordell, *Introduction to Alkaloids* (New York, Wiley-Interscience, 1981).

11. Black, *Folk-Medicine*, p. 194.

12. Mrs M. Grieve, *A Modern Herbal* (London, Jonathan Cape, 1931), p. 577.

13. J.A. Duke, *Handbook of Medicinal Herbs* (Boca Raton, Florida, CRC Press, 1985).

14. National Library of Scotland, MS3774.

15. F. Marian McNeill, *The Scots Kitchen* (London, Blackie, 1929), p. 93.

16. Alexander Carmichael, *Carmina Gadelica*, 6 vols (Edinburgh, 1900–71), vol. V, p. 125.

17. Mr A.E.R., personal communication (Northampton, 1985).

18. Dr Speller claims 'there is little in these bizarre and entertaining "cures" that can have any basis in therapeutics.' (See also n. 2 above.) Letter in Margaret Baker, *Folklore and Customs of Rural England* (Newton Abbott, Devon, David & Charles, 1974), p. 169. Another author goes so far as to state, 'In general, native plant

remedies are of little value', D.J. Guthrie, *Transactions of the Botanical Society of Edinburgh*, 1961, vol. 39, part II.

19. N. Culpeper, *The English Physician* (London, 1652).
20. E.P. Thompson, *Customs in Common* (Suffolk, Merlin Press, 1981).
21. George Ewart Evans, *Where Beards Wag All* (London, Faber & Faber, 1970), p. 18.
22. I. Hirono *et al*, 'Carcinogenic activity of *Symphytum officinale*', *Journal of the National Cancer Institute*, 1978, 61: 865–9.
23. E.B., d.o.b. *c.*1930, personal communication (Cheshire, 1985).
24. J. Brauchli *et al.*, 'Pyrrolizidine alkaloids from *Symphytum officinale* L. and their percutaneous absorption in rats', *Experientia* 1982, 38: 1085–7.
25. P.C. Anderson and A.E.M. McLean, 'Comfrey and liver damage', *Human Toxicology*, 1989, 8: 55–74.
26. Mr R.H. Eriswell, d.o.b. *c.*1920, personal communication (Suffolk, 1987).
27. Toftwood School, Norfolk, 1988.
28. Mrs A.H.S., d.o.b. *c.*1945, personal communication (Aylsham, Norfolk, 1992).
29. Unpublished project: Mundford Primary School, Norfolk, 1980.
30. Mr D.E.B., d.o.b. 1925; Age Concern Essay (Chelmsford, Essex, 1991).
31. Logan Home Papers (Scottish Records Office, GDI 384/26).
32. Grieve, *A Modern Herbal*, p. 655.
33. L.F. Newman and E.M. Wilson, 'Folklore survivals in the southern "Lake Counties" and in Essex: a Comparison and Contrast', *Folklore* 1951, 62: 252–66.
34. Grieve, *A Modern Herbal*, p. 193.
35. Numerous records, e.g. Mr W.G., d.o.b. *c.*1910, personal communication (Witton, Norfolk, 1988).
36. Mr J.C., d.o.b. 1907, personal communication (Stowbridge, Norfolk, 1996).
37. Mrs M.B., d.o.b. *c.*1930, personal communication (Great Yarmouth, Norfolk, 1988).
38. Mrs G., d.o.b. *c.*1930, personal communication (Hemsby, Norfolk, 1988).
39. Mr J., personal commmunication (Witton, Norfolk, 1988).
40. Mrs G., d.o.b. *c.*1930, personal communication (Hemsby, Norfolk, 1988).

41. R.C. Wren, *Potter's New Cyclopaedia of Botanical Drugs and Preparations*, completely revised by E.M. Williamson and F.J. Evans (Saffron Walden, C.W. Daniel Co., 1988), p. 226.

42. Mr M., d.o.b. 1935, personal communication (Wymondham, Norfolk, 1987).

43. Blythburgh W.I., Suffolk, *c.*1920 recorded by Dr Mark Taylor (Norfolk Records Office MS4322).

44. Mr G., d.o.b. 1900, personal communication (Ludham, Norfolk, 1988).

45. Black, *Folk-Medicine*, p. 191.

46. Ibid., p. 135.

47. Grieve, *A Modern Herbal*, p. 831.

48. The Revd T.O. Cockayne, 1864, *Leechdoms, Wortcunning and Starcraft of Early England*, 3 vols (London, Holland Press, 1961), vol. I, p. 91.

49. Ibid.

50. John Gerard, *The Herball or Generall Historie of Plantes* (London, 1597).

51. John M. Riddle, *Quid Pro Quo: Studies in the History of Drugs* (Hampshire, Variorum Press, Ashgate Publishing Ltd, 1992), p. 164.

52. D.E. Nagy, *Popular Medicine in Seventeenth-Century England* (Ohio, Bowling Green State University Popular Press, 1988), p. 73.

53. Riddle, *Quid Pro Quo*, p. 165.

54. Malcolm Stuart (ed.), *The Encyclopaedia of Herbs and Herbalism* (London, Orbis, 1979), p. 10.

55. Charles Singer, *From Magic to Science* (London, Dover Publications, 1958), p. 169.

56. Charles Singer, Introduction, *Leechdoms, Wortcunning and Starcraft of Early England*, ed. Revd T. Cockayne (London, Holland Press, 1961), p. xli.

57. Ernest R. Suffling, *History and Legends of the Broads District* (Norwich, Jarrold, 1891), p. 87.

58. Mrs A.E., d.o.b. *c.*1945, personal communication (Whissonsett, Norfolk, 1988).

59. Tony Hunt, *Popular Medicine in Thirteenth Century England* (Woodbridge, Brewer, 1990), Chapter V.

60. John M. Riddle, *Contraception and Abortion from the Ancient World to the Renaissance* (Harvard University Press, 1992), pp. 91, 106.

61. Ibid., p. 155.

62. This interpretation of the doctrine of signatures was first suggested to me by a medical herbalist in 1984, and I have since

seen it hinted at elsewhere, e.g. by Richard Mabey in his recent *Flora Britannica* (1996), where on p. 300, writing about the doctrine of signatures, he says 'sometimes it seems to have been a form of aide-memoire'.

63. John Pechey, *The Compleat Herbal of Physical Plants* (London, 1694), p. 164.
64. Miss H.C. Colman, *Princes Street Magazine*, November 1924, p. 173.
65. Leven and Melville Papers, 1661–1702 (Scottish Records Office, GD 26/6/207).
66. Mrs L.M.H., Age Concern essay (Colchester, Essex, 1991).
67. Pechey, *The Compleat Herbal*, Preface.
68. Evans, *Where Beards Wag All*, p. 18.
69. G. Hatfield, *Warts: A Report of a Survey for the Folklore Society* (University College London, Folklore Society, 1998).
70. See Chapter 6 of this book.

Chapter 4: The People Themselves: The Users of Domestic Medicine

1. Mr George G., personal communication (Ludham, Norfolk, 1989).
2. Mrs Vera W., personal communication (Brundall, Norfolk, 1989).
3. Mrs D., personal communication (Horning, Norfolk, 1989).
4. Mr W. A., personal communication (Trunch, Norfolk, 1989).
5. Mrs J., personal communication (Salhouse, Norfolk, 1990).
6. Mr G., d.o.b. *c.*1920, personal communication (Brundall, Norfolk, 1989).
7. Mrs G., d.o.b. *c.*1920, personal communication (Hemsby, Norfolk, 1989).
8. Mr B., d.o.b. *c.*1905, personal communication (Horning, Norfolk, 1989); Mundford Primary School, school project on family cures, collected in the 1980s. *See also* Enid Porter, *The Folklore of East Anglia* (London, Batsford, 1974).
9. Mrs A.M., personal communication (Wakefield, West Yorkshire, 1985).
10. Geoffrey Grigson, *The Englishman's Flora* (London, Phoenix House, 1955), p. 216.

11. Mrs E.D., personal communication (Taunton, Somerset, 1985).
12. E.J.C., unpublished Age Concern essay (Wickford, Essex, 1991).
13. Mrs B., unpublished Age Concern essay (Essex, 1991).
14. Mrs E.F., unpublished Age Concern essay (Great Waltham, Essex, 1991).
15. Mrs E.M., d.o.b. 1917, unpublished Age Concern essay (St Osyth, Essex, 1991).
16. Mrs B.B., unpublished Essex Age Concern essay (Southend-on-Sea, Essex, 1991).
17. Mrs M.W., unpublished Age Concern essay (Saffron Waldon, Essex, 1991).
18. Mrs D.T., d.o.b. *c.*1910, personal communication (Rockland St Mary, Norfolk, 1990).
19. Mrs A.P., personal communication (Moulton, Norfolk, 1989).
20. Mr D.H., personal communication (Lowestoft, Suffolk, 1988).
21. Mrs A., personal communication (North Walsham, Norfolk, 1990).
22. Porter, *The Folklore of East Anglia*, p. 42.
23. Frederick C. Wigby, *Just a Country Boy* (Wymondham, Norfolk, Geo R. Reeve Ltd., 1976).
24. F.C. Wigby, personal commmunication (Norwich, June 1990).
25. Wigby, *Just A Country Boy*.
26. F.C. Wigby, personal communication (Norwich, June 1990).
27. Marcus Woodward (ed.), *Gerard's Herball. The Essence thereof distilled by Marcus Woodward from the edition of Th Johnson, 1636* (London, Howe, 1927), p. 201.
28. Wigby, *Just a Country Boy*, p. 65.
29. *Gerard's Herball*, p. 62.
30. Wigby, *Just a Country Boy*, p. 65.
31. *Gerard's Herball*, p. 88.
32. Wigby, *Just a Country Boy*, p. 65.
33. *Gerard's Herball*, p. 189.
34. Wigby, *Just a Country Boy*, p. 65.
35. *Gerard's Herball*, p. 83.
36. Agnes Arber, *Herbals: Their Origin and Evolution* (London, Jonathan Cape, 1939), p. 270.
37. Mrs L.M.H., Essex Age Concern essay (Colchester, Essex, 1991).
38. Gervase Markham, *The English Housewife* (9th edition, London, 1688).
39. Roy Porter, *Disease, Medicine and Society in England, 1550–1860* (second edition, Cambridge University Press, 1995), p. 3.
40. 'Life of Adam Donald', *The Bee* (Dec 21, 1791).

41. M. Muncaster 'Medical Services and the Medical Profession in Norfolk 1815–1911', 2 vols (Ph.D. thesis, University of East Anglia, 1976), vol. I, p. 207.

42. Dr Mark R. Taylor, manuscript notes (Norfolk Records Office, MS 4322, 57x1).

43. See G. Hatfield, 'Domestic Medicine in Eighteenth Century Scotland' (Ph.D. thesis, University of Edinburgh, 1980), p. 105.

44. Clerk of Penicuik Papers (Scottish Records Office, GD18/2142).

45. Roy Palmer, *Britain's Living Folklore* (David & Charles, 1991), p. 144.

46. Quoted in Dr N. Gunn, *The Book of Linton Church* (Peebles, Neidpath Press, 1912), p. 84.

47. John Pechey, *Compleat Herbal of Physical Plants* (London, 1694), p. 176.

48. Mrs M. Grieve, *A Modern Herbal* (Jonathan Cape, 1931), p. 500.

49. Roy Vickery, *A Dictionary of Plant Lore* (Oxford University Press, 1995), p. 358.

50. *Notes and Sketches illustrative of Northern Rural Life in the Eighteenth Century by the Author of Johnny Gibb of Gushetneuk* (Edinburgh, Douglas, 1877).

51. Miss N., now resident in Norfolk, personal communication (Norfolk, 1989)

52. Vickery, *A Dictionary of Plant Lore*, p. 357.

53. Tess Darwin, *The Scots Herbal* (Edinburgh, Mercat Press, 1996), p. 76.

54. See e.g. Vickery, *Dictionary of Plant Lore*, p. 108.

55. Roger Frith, 'Old Remedies and Charms of Essex', *East Anglian Magazine*, June 1965, p. 284.

56. Mr H., personal communication (Lowestoft, 1990).

57. *Gunton Household Book* (Church of St Peter Mancroft, Norwich).

58. Dolly Rafter MS (privately owned).

Chapter 5: Magic and Medicine

1. E.P. Thompson, *Customs in Common* (Suffolk, Merlin Press, 1991), p. 21.

2. G.L. Gomme, *Encyclopedia of Religion and Ethics* (Edinburgh, 1913), pp. 57–9.

3.   See R. Porter, *Disease, Medicine and Society in England* (Cambridge University Press, 1995), p. 3.

4.   Thompson, *Customs in Common*, p. 17.

5.   George Ewart Evans, *Where Beards Wag All* (London, Faber & Faber, 1970), p. 21.

6.   See e.g. George Ewart Evans, *The Days That We Have Seen* (London, Faber & Faber, 1975), p. 29ff.

7.   F. Marian McNeil, *The Scots Kitchen* (London, Blackie, 1929), p. 93.

8.   James Mason, 'The Folklore of British Plants', *Dublin University Magazine*, November 1873, p. 558.

9.   Ibid., p. 555.

10.   Dorothy Porter and Roy Porter, *Patient's Progress: Doctors and Doctoring in Eighteenth Century England* (Cambridge, Polity Press, 1989), p. 35.

11.   Mr D.H.C., Age Concern essay (Boxted, Essex, 1990).

12.   J. and E. Brooke, *Suffolk Prospect* (London, Faber & Faber, 1963), p. 105.

13.   Lilias Rider Haggard (ed.), *I Walked by Night* (Woodbridge, Boydell Press, 1974), p. 16.

14.   *Gerard's Herball. The essence thereof distilled by Marcus Woodward from the edition of Th. Johnson, 1636.* (London, Howe, 1927), p. 94.

15.   Mrs I.H., personal communication (Norfolk, 1989).

16.   Scottish Records Office (Edinburgh, SRO GD 18/5219). Quoted by Rosalind K. Marshall in *Childhood in Seventeenth Century Scotland* (Edinburgh, Trustees of the National Gallery of Scotland, 1976).

17.   Peter Buchan, *Ancient Ballads and Songs of the North of Scotland*, 2 vols (Edinburgh, 1828), vol. II, p. 39.

18.   Letter from Mrs Campbell, of the house of Breadalabane, writing to Lady Breadalbane in 1778. Quoted in Marion Lochhead, *The Scots Household in the Eighteenth Century* (Edinburgh, Moray Press, 1948), p. 338.

19.   Mrs S.W., d.o.b. *c.*1955, personal communication (Suffolk,1989).

20.   *Notes from Diary of George Ridpath, Minister of Stitchel, 1755–1761.* Edited with Notes and Introduction by Sir James Balfour Paul (Edinburgh, printed by Constable for Scottish History Society, 1922).

21.   *Gerard's Herball*, p. 109.

22.   National Library of Scotland, MS 3774.

23.   *Gunton Household Book* (Norwich, Church of St Peter Mancroft).

24. Ibid. China roots is probably a species of *Smilax*.
25. Ibid.
26. Recipe and prescription book of (?) Elizabeth, wife of the fourth Lord Walsingham (Norfolk Records Office, LXIV/35).
27. Sir John Cullum's copy of *Flora Anglica* (W. Hudson, 1762). The copy is in the West Suffolk Records Office, and is annotated by Sir James Cullum. This information apppears on p. 163.
28. West Suffolk Records Office, *Philosophical Letters Between the late learned Mr Ray and several of his Ingenious Correspondents* (London, 1718).
29. Cullum, *Flora Angelica*, see n. 27.
30. *Gunton Household Book.*
31. William Buchan, *Domestic Medicine: or a Treatise on the Prevention and Cure of Diseases by Regimen and Simple Medicines* (Glasgow, 1806).
32. The Revd J. Wesley's book *Primitive Physic*, 1755 edition, formed the basis of William H. Paynter (ed.), *Primitive Physic. A Book of Old Fashioned Cures and Remedies* (8th edn, 1982), Preface.
33. Jolande Jacobi (ed.), *Paracelsus. Selected Writings* (London, Routledge & Kegan Paul, 1951), p. 199.
34. Richard Sanders (Student in the Divine and Celestial Sciences), *Physiognomie, and Chiromancie, Metoscopie, The Symmetrical Proportions and Signal Moles of the Body, Fully and accurately handled; with their Natural – Predictive – Significations* (London, 1653).
35. Quoted in Agnes Arber, *Herbals: Their Origin and Evolution* (2nd edn, Cambridge University Press, 1953), p. 254.
36. Leon Petulengro, *Romany Boy* (London, Robert Hale, 1979), p. 21.
37. Keith Thomas, *Religion and the Decline of Magic* (Harmondsworth, Penguin, 1973), p. 196.
38. Mrs F., personal communication (Loddon, Norfolk, 1988).
39. C.P. Petch and E.L. Swann, *Flora of Norfolk* (Norwich, Jarrold, 1968), p. 168.
40. S. Drury, 'Herbal Remedies for livestock in Seventeenth and Eighteenth Century England: Some Examples', *Folklore*, 96, ii, 1985, pp. 243–7.
41. Susan M. Palliser, *The Use of Plants in English Folk Medicine* (Leeds Folklore Group, School of English, University of Leeds, 1984).
42. Mary Beith, *Healing Threads* (Polygon, Edinburgh, 1995).
43. Derek Bryce (ed.), *The Herbal Remedies of the Physicians of Myddfai*, trans. John Pugh (Lampeter, Llanerch, 1987).

44. See e.g. Charles McGlinchey, *The Last of the Name*, Brian Friel
     (ed.) (Belfast, Blackstaff Press, 1986), p. 83ff.
45. 'The Workes of ... Mr William Pemble' (3rd edition, 1635), p.
     559, quoted in Keith Thomas, *Religion and the Decline of Magic*
     (Harmondsworth, Penguin, 1973), p. 194.
46. E.P., 'The Winnowing of White Witchcraft' (British Museum MS
     Sloane, 1954).
47. Reginald Scott, *Discoverie*, quoted in Keith Thomas, *Religion and
     the Decline of Magic*, p. 518.
48. Ibid., p. 226.
49. Mrs L.M.H., Age Concern essay (Colchester, Essex, 1990).

Chapter 6: Warts and All

1.   See Roy Vickery, *A Dictionary of Plant Lore* (Oxford University
     Press, 1995), p. 383.
2.   Numerous records, e.g. Mrs E., personal communication
     (Norwich, 1989); *see also* R. Vickery, 'The use of Broad Beans to
     cure Warts', *Folklore*, vol. 102 (ii), 1991, pp. 239–40.
3.   English Folklore Survey (unpublished), Dorset, M172 West
     Country M6: Hants M52.
4.   English Folklore Survey (unpublished), Norfolk M72; Dorset
     M100.
5.   See G. Hatfield, *Warts: Summary of Wart-cure Survey for the
     Folklore Society* (London, Folklore Society, 1998).
6.   English Folklore Survey (University College London, 1960s,
     unpublished), Wilts M189.
7.   Kevin Danaher, *The Year in Ireland. Irish Calendar Customs* (Dublin,
     Mercier Publications, 1994).
8.   E.L. Mishenkova *et al.*, 'Antiviral properties of St John's Wort and
     preparations produced from it', *Tr S'ezda Mikrobiol Ukr* 1975,
     pp. 222–3.
9.   For example, the greater celandine, (*Chelidonium majus*), see *U.S.
     Dispensatory* 25, 1623.
10. M.J.U. Ferreira, A.M. Lobo, H. Wyler, 'Triterpenoids and Steroids
     from Euphorbia peplus', *Fitoterapia* 64(1): 85–7 (1993).
11. H. Itokawa, Y. Ichihara, K. Watanabe, K. Takeya, 'An Antitumor
     principle from Euphorbia lathyris', *Planta Medica* 55(3): 272
     (1989).

12.	Andrew Chevalier, *The Encyclopedia of Medicinal Plants* (London, Dorling Kindersley, 1996).
13.	English Folklore Survey (unpublished).
14.	Hatfield, *Warts. Summary of Wart-cure Survey*, p. 18.
15.	Chevalier, *The Encyclopedia of Medicinal Plants*, p. 185.
16.	John Moncrief, *The Poor Man's Physician* (3rd edn, Edinburgh, 1731).
17.	Susan M. Palliser, *Plants as Wart Cures in Seventeenth and Eighteenth Century England* (Leeds, Leeds Folklore Group, School of English, 1983).
18.	Hatfield, *Warts. Summary of Wart-cure Survey*, p. 4.
19.	J.A. Marshall and E.C.M. Haes, *Grasshoppers and allied insects of Great Britain and Ireland* (Colchester, Harley Books, 1988), pp. 82–4.
20.	Letter from F.P. (unpublished) (Great Yarmouth, 1963; English Folklore Survey, M72).
21.	Ibid.
22.	English Folklore Survey (unpublished), M174.
23.	Mr O., personal communication, (Brundall, Norfolk, 1990).
24.	Mr D.R.T., personal communication, (Caston, Norfolk, 1997).
25.	Mr J.K., personal communication, (Norfolk, 1989).
26.	Letter to Mark R. Taylor from B.J. and H.L.B., Heacham (Norfolk Records Office, MS4322).
27.	D.M. Ewin, 'Hypnotherapy for Warts', *American Journal of Clinical Hypnosis* 35(1), July 1992, pp. 1–10.
28.	N.W., personal communication (Norwich, 1996).
29.	Jane Sterling, 'Treating the Troublesome Wart', in *The Practitioner* (January 1995), vol. 239, pp. 44–7.
30.	K. Steele, 'Wart charming practices among patients attending wart clinics', *British Journal of General Practice*, December 1990, pp. 517–18.
31.	D.A. Burns, 'Warts and all – the history and folklore of warts: a review', *Journal of the Royal Society of Medicine*, 85, January 1992, pp. 37–40.
32.	Milton S. Ross, 'Warts in the Medical Folklore of Europe', *International Journal of Dermatology*, 18 (1979), pp. 505–9.
33.	English Folklore Survey, M171.
34.	D.A. Burns, 'Warts and all'.
35.	See Vickery, *A Dictionary of Plant Lore*.

Chapter 7: Hedgerow or Herb Patch: Sources of Plants used in Domestic Medicine

1. Mr W.G., personal communication (Witton, Norfolk, 1988).
2. Mrs G., personal communication (Hemsby, Norfolk, 1988).
3. Mrs V.W., personal communication (Brundall, Norfolk, 1988).
4. *Gunton Household Book* (Norwich, Church of St Peter Mancroft).
5. See Roy Vickery, *A Dictionary of Plant Lore* (Oxford University Press, 1995), p. 337.
6. John Pechey, *The Compleat Herbal of Physical Plants* (London, 1694).
7. William Alexander, *Notes and Sketches Illustrative of Northern Rural Life in the Eighteenth Century by the Author of Johnny Gibb of Gushetneuk* (Edinburgh, David Douglas, 1877), p. 12.
8. M. Grieve, *A Modern Herbal* (London, Jonathan Cape, 1931), p. 536.
9. Tess Darwin, *The Scots Herbal* (Edinburgh, Mercat Press, 1996), p. 95.
10. Bea Howe, *Lady with Green Fingers* (London, Country Life, 1961), p. 18.
11. M.R. Mitford, *Our Village* (London, Whittaker, 1824).
12. Quoted in Geoffrey Grigson, *The Englishman's Flora* (London, Phoenix House, 1955), p. 316.
13. Mary Webb, *The Golden Arrow* (London, Jonathan Cape, 1916), p. 176.
14. Roger Frith, 'Old Remedies and Charms of Essex', *East Anglian Magazine*, June 1965, p. 284.
15. Mrs D.T., d.o.b. 1908, personal communication (Rockland St Mary, Norfolk, 1988); Mrs P.B., d.o.b. *c.*1940, personal communication (Norwich, 1989).
16. Doris Coates, *Tuppeny Rice and Treacle. Cottage Housekeeping 1900–1920* (Newton Abbott, Devon, David & Charles, 1975).
17. Mrs B., Age Concern essay (Essex, 1991).
18. Mrs M.S., d.o.b. 1914, Age Concern essay (Essex, 1991).
19. Mrs E.F., d.o.b. 1902, Age Concern essay (Essex, 1991).
20. D.E. Allen, MS.
21. Mrs M.B., d.o.b. *c.*1930, personal communication (Great Yarmouth, 1988).
22. Mrs M.M, personal communication (Wiltshire, 1998).
23. Mr. M., personal communication (Wymondham, 1989).

24. Quoted in Grieve, *A Modern Herbal*, p. 442.

25. *Norfolk and Norwich Notes and Queries*, vol. I, 1905–1915, answer to query no. 544.

26. Grieve, *A Modern Herbal*, p. 820. Dr Thornton himself used Tormentil in the treatment of fluxes of blood.

27. Charles McGlinchey, *The Last of the Name*, Brian Friel (ed.) (Belfast, Blackstaff Press, 1986).

28. *Mrs Lavender's Herbal Book* (London, Shurey's Publications Ltd., n.d.), p. 4.

29. See statistics in Hatfield, *Country Remedies* (Woodbridge, Boydell Press, 1994), p. 77.

Chapter 8: Old Cures, New Healing: The Effectiveness of Plant Remedies

1. C.A. Newall, L.A. Anderson, J.D. Phillipson, *Herbal Medicines. A Guide for Health-care Professionals* (London, The Pharmaceutical Press, 1996).

2. John M. Riddle, *Contraception and Abortion from the Ancient World to the Renaissance* (Harvard University Press, 1992).

3. E.S. Johnson *et al.*, 1985, *British Medical Journal*, 291: 569.

4. Mrs M.S., d.o.b. 1914, Essex Age Concern essay (Braintree, Essex, 1990).

5. Ibid.

6. See e.g. M. Wainwright, 'Moulds in Medicine', *Folklore*, 100 (ii): 162–6 (1989).

7. Mrs E.M., d.o.b. 1917, Essex Age Concern essay (St Osyth, Essex, 1990).

8. Laura Hastings, 'The Botanic Gardens at Kew and the Wartime Need for Medicines', *The Pharmaceutical Journal*, 257: 923–7 (1996).

9. C.E. Hennels, 'The Wild Herb Men', *East Anglian Magazine*, December 1972, pp. 79–80.

10. See article by Lucy Pinney, in *The Times Weekend*, Saturday June 26 1999, pp. 1–2.

BIBLIOGRAPHY

Arber, A., *Herbals, their Origin and Evolution*, 2nd edn (Cambridge University Press, 1953)

Aubrey, J., *The Natural History of Wiltshire*, ed. J. Britten (London, 1847)

Baker, M., *Folklore and Customs of Rural England* (Devon, David & Charles, 1974)

Beith, M., *Healing Threads* (Edinburgh, Polygon, 1995)

Black. W.G., *Folk-Medicine* (London, Folklore Society, 1883)

Bonnard, B., *Channel Island Plant Lore* (Guernsey Press, 1993)

British Pharmaceutical Codex (London, Pharmaceutical Press, 1923)

Broome, A.S., *Bob's Boy*, ed. David Poole (Norwich, Wilson-Poole, 1984)

Bryant, C., *Flora Dietetica* (London, 1783)

Buchan, P., *Ancient Ballads and Songs of the North of Scotland*, 2 vols (Edinburgh, 1828)

Buchan, W., *Domestic Medicine* (Glasgow, 1806)

Bynum, W.F. and Porter, R. (eds), *Medical Fringe and Medical Orthodoxy 1750–1850* (London, Croom Helm, 1986)

Carmichael, A., *Carmina Gadelica*, 6 vols (Edinburgh, 1900–71)

Chevalier, A., *The Encylopedia of Medicinal Plants* (London, Dorling Kindersley, 1996)

Child, F.J., *English and Scottish Popular Ballads*, 8 vols (Boston, 1857–9)

Coates, D., *Tuppeny Rice and Treacle* (Devon, David & Charles, 1975)

Cockayne, Revd T.O., *Leechdoms, Wortcunning and Starcraft of Early England*, 1864 (London, Holland Press, 1961)

Coles, W., *Adam in Eden* (J. Streater for Nathaniel Brooke, London, 1657)

Cordell, G.A., *Introduction to Alkaloids* (New York, Wiley-Interscience, 1981)

Culpeper, N., *The English Physician* (London, 1652)

Danaher, *The Year in Ireland* (Dublin, Mercier Publications, 1994)

Darwin, T., *The Scots Herbal* (Edinburgh, Mercat Press, 1996)

Defoe, D., *A Tour through the Whole Island of Great Britain*, 4 vols (London, 1753)

Duke, J.A., *The Green Pharmacy* (Pennsylvania, Rodale Press, 1997)

Duke, J.A., *Handbook of Medicinal Herbs* (Boca Raton, Florida, CRC Press, 1985)

Emerson, P.H., *Pictures of East Anglian Life* (London, Sampson, Low, Marston, Searle & Rittington, 1888)

Evans, G.E., *The Pattern under the Plough* (London, Faber & Faber, 1966)

Evans, G.E., *The Horse in the Furrow* (London, Faber & Faber, 1960)

Evans, G.E., *Where Beards Wag All* (London, Faber & Faber, 1970)

Evans, G.E., *The Days that We Have Seen* (London, Faber & Faber, 1975)

French, C.N., (ed.), *A Countryman's Day Book* (London, J.M. Dent & Sons, 1929)

Gardiner J. and N. Wenborn (eds), *British History* (London, Collins & Brown, 1995)

Geertz, C., *Local Knowledge* (London, Hutchinson, 1993)

Gerard, J., *The Herball or Generall Historie of Plantes* (London, 1597)

Gomme, G.L., *Encyclopedia of Religion and Ethics* (Edinburgh, 1913)

Grieve, Mrs M., *A Modern Herbal* (London, Jonathan Cape, 1931)

Griggs, B., *Green Pharmacy* (London, Jill Norman & Hobhouse, 1981)

Grigson, G., *The Englishman's Flora* (London, Phoenix House, 1955)

Gunn, Dr N., *The Book of Linton Church* (Peebles, Neidpath Press, 1912)

Harvey, A.S., *Ballads, Songs and Rhymes of East Anglia* (Norwich, Jarrold, 1936)

Hatfield, G., *Country Remedies* (Woodbridge, Boydell Press, 1994)

Hatfield, G., *Warts, Summary of Wart Cure Survey* (London, Foklore Society, 1999)

Howe, B., *Lady with Green Fingers* (London, Country Life, 1961)

Hudson, W., *Flora Anglica* (London, 1762)

Hunt, T., *Popular Medicine in Thirteenth Century Britain* (Cambrige, Brewer, 1990)

Hunt, T., *Plant Names of Medieval England* (Cambridge, Brewer, 1989)

Jacobi, J. (ed.), *Paracelsus, Selected Writings* (London, Routledge & Kegan Paul, 1951)

Jamieson, J., *A Dictionary of the Scottish Language*, 4 vols (Edinburgh University Press, 1808)

Lafonte, A.M., *Herbal Folklore* (Bideford, Badger Books, 1984)

Lavender, *Mrs Lavender's Herbal Book* (London, Shurey Publications, n.d.)

Lawson, A., *The Modern Farrier* (London, 1842)

Leyel, Mrs C.F., *The Magic of Herbs* (London, Jonathan Cape, 1926)

Mabey, R., *Flora Britannica* (London, Sinclair-Stevenson, 1996)

Mardle, J., *Norfolk Characters* (Norwich, George Nobbs, 1976)

Markam, G., *The English Housewife*, 9th edn (London, 1688)

Marshall, J.A. and E.C.M. Haes, *Grasshoppers and Allied Insects of Great Britain and Ireland* (Colchester, Harley Books, 1988)

Marshall, R.K., *Childhood in Seventeenth Century Scotland* (Edinburgh, Trustees of the National Gallery of Scotland, 1976)

McGlinchey, C., *The Last of the Name*, ed. Brian Friel (Belfast, Blackstaff Press, 1986)

McNeill, F.M., *The Scots Kitchen* (London, Blackie, 1929)

Medical Botany or History of Plants in the Materia Medica of the London, Edinburgh and Dublin Pharmacopoeias (London, 1819)

Mitford, M.R., *Our Village* (London, Wittaker, 1824)

Morton, A.G., *History of Botanical Science* (London, Academic Press, 1981)

Nagy, D.E., Newall, C.A., Anderson, Linda A., Phillipson, David J., *Popular Medicine in Seventeenth Century England* (Ohio, Bowling Green State University Popular Press, 1988)

Notes and Sketches Illustrative of Northern Rural (Edinburgh, Douglas, 1877)

Nuttall, G.C., *Wild Flowers as they Grow* (London, Waverley Book Company., n.d.)

Palmer, R., *Britain's Living Folklore* (Devon, David & Charles, 1991)

Paynter, W.H. (ed.), *John Wesley, Primitive Physic*, 8th edn (Cornwall, 1982)

Pechey, J., *The Compleat Herbal of Physical Plants* (London, 1694)

Pennant, T., *A Tour in Scotland 1769* (London, 1776)

Pennecuik, A., *Description of Tweeddale* (Leith, 1815)

Perkin, J., *Victorian Women* (London, Murray, 1993)

Petch, C.P. and E.L. Swann, *Flora of Norfolk* (Norwich, Jarrold, 1968)

Petulengro, L., *Romany Boy* (London, Robert Hale, 1979)

Phillipson, D., *Herbal Medicines* (London, Pharmaceutical Press, 1996)

Pigott, B.A.F., *Flowers and Ferns of Cromer and its Neighbourhood* (Norwich, Jarrold, 1882)

Pococke, R., Bishop of Meath, *Tours in Scotland, 1747, 1750, 1760*, ed. D.W. Kemp (Edinburgh University Press; printed by Constable for the Scottish History Society, 1887)

Porter, D. and Porter, R., *Patient's Progress: Doctors and Doctoring in Eighteenth Century England* (Cambridge, Polity Press, 1989)

Porter, E., *The Folklore of East Anglia* (London, Batsford, 1974)

Porter, R., *Disease, Medicine and Society in England, 1550–1860*, second edn (Cambridge University Press, 1995)

Porter, R., *England in the Eighteenth Century* (London, Folio Society, 1998)

Pratt, A., *Wild Flowers* (London, 1898)

Quiller-Couch, Sir A. (ed.), *The Oxford Book of English Verse* (Oxford University Press, 1939)

Rider Haggard, L. (ed.), *I Walked by Night* (Woodbridge, Boydell Press, 1974)

Riddle, J.M., *Eve's Herbs: A History of Contraception and Abortion in the West* (Harvard University Press, 1997)

Riddle, J.M., *Contraception and Abortion from the Ancient World to the Renaissance* (Harvard University Press, 1992)

Riddle, J.M., *Quid Pro Quo: Studies in the History of Drugs* (Hampshire, Variorum Press, Ashgate Publishing, 1992)

Ridpath, G., *Diary of George Ridpath, Minister of Stitchel 1755–1761*, ed. Sir James Balfour (Edinburgh, printed by Constable for the Scottish History Society, 1922)

Sachs, J. von, *History of Botany*, transl. H.E.F. Garnsey (Oxford, Clarendon Press, 1890)

Salmon, W., *The Compleat English Physician* (London, 1693)

Saunders, R., *Physiognomie, and Chiromancie, Metocopie, The Symmetrical Proportions and Signal Moles of the Body, Fully and accurately handled, with their Natural – Predictive – Significations* (London, 1653)

Singer, C., *From Magic to Science* (London, Dover Publications, 1958)

Skargon, Y., *A Calendar of Herbs* (Scolar Press, 1978)

Smith, J.C. and de Selincourt, E., (eds), *Spenser: Complete Poetical Works* (Oxford Unversity Press, 1912)

Stearn, W.T., *Botanical Latin* (London, Nelson, 1966)

Suffling, E.R., *History and Legends of the Broads District* (Norwich, Jarrold, 1891)

Thomas, K., *Religion and the Decline of Magic* (Harmondsworth, Penguin, 1973)

Thompson, E.P., *Customs in Common* (Harmondsworth, Penguin, 1993)

Thompson, F.M.L. (ed.), *The Cambridge Social History of Britain*, 3 vols (Cambridge University Press, 1990)

Trevelyan, G.M., *England under the Stuarts* (London, Folio Society, 1946)

Turner, W., *The first and second parts of the Herbal ... with the third parte* (London, 1568)

Turner, W., *Libellus de Re Herbaria 1538 and The Names of Herbes 1548* (Ray Society, London, 1965)

Vickery, R., *A Dictionary of Plant Lore* (Oxford University Press, 1995)

Webb, M., *The Golden Arrow* (London, Jonathan Cape, 1916)

Wigby, F.C., *Just a Country Boy* (Wymondham. Geo.R. Reeve, 1976)

Woodward, M. (ed.), *Gerard's Herball: The essence thereof distilled by Marcus Woodward* (London, Howe, 1927)

Wren, R.C., *Potter's New Cyclopaedia of Botanical Drugs and Preparations* (Devon, Health Science Press, 1975)

Wren, R.C., *Potter's New Cyclopedia of Botanical Drugs and Preparations* (Saffron Walden, C.W. Daniel Co., 1988)

Young, J., *Farming in East Anglia* (London, David Rendel, 1967)

Zamoyska, B., *The Burston Rebellion* (London, BBC, 1985)

GENERAL INDEX

Numbers in **bold** indicate illustrations

INDEX TO PLANT NAMES

The names quoted for British plant names are in accordance with C. Stace, *New Flora of the British Isles* (Cambridge University Press, 1991). Others are in accordance with D.J. Mabberley, *The Plant-Book* (Cambridge University Press, 1987).

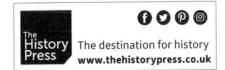

ALSO FROM THE HISTORY PRESS

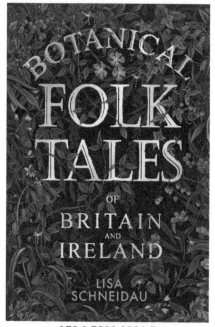

978 0 7509 8121 7

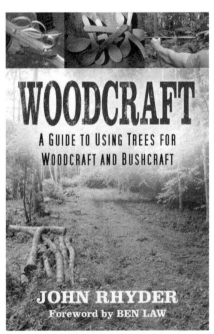

WOODCRAFT

A Guide to Using Trees for Woodcraft and Bushcraft

JOHN RHYDER
Foreword by BEN LAW

978 0 7509 9818 5